The 11–14-week scan

The diagnosis of fetal abnormalities

Dedication

To
Herodotos and Despina

Diploma in Fetal Medicine Series
Series Editor: K. H. Nicolaides

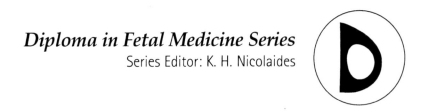

The 11–14-week scan

The diagnosis of fetal abnormalities

Kypros H. Nicolaides,
Neil J. Sebire & Rosalinde J. M. Snijders

The Parthenon Publishing Group
International Publishers in Medicine, Science & Technology

NEW YORK   LONDON

Library of Congress Cataloging-in-Publication Data
Data available on request

British Library Cataloguing in Publication Data
Data available on request

ISBN 1-85070-743-X
ISSN 1467-2162

Published in the USA by
The Parthenon Publishing Group Inc.
One Blue Hill Plaza
Pearl River
New York 10965, USA

Published in the UK and Europe by
The Parthenon Publishing Group Ltd.
Casterton Hall, Carnforth
Lancs. LA6 2LA, UK

Copyright 1999 © Parthenon Publishing Group

First published 1999

Typeset by AMA DataSet Ltd., Preston, UK
Printed and bound by Butler & Tanner Ltd., Frome and London, UK

Contents

Introduction

In 1866, Langdon Down reported that the skin of individuals with trisomy 21 appears to be too large for their body. In the 1990s, it was realized that the excess skin of individuals with Down's syndrome can be visualized by ultrasonography as increased nuchal translucency in the first 3 months of intrauterine life. Fetal nuchal translucency thickness at the 11–14-week scan has been combined with maternal age to provide an effective method of screening for trisomy 21; for an invasive testing rate of 5%, about 75% of trisomic pregnancies can be identified. When maternal serum free-β human chorionic gonadotropin and pregnancy-associated plasma protein-A at 11–14 weeks are also taken into account, the detection rate of chromosomal defects is about 90%.

In addition to its role in the assessment of risk for trisomy 21, increased nuchal translucency thickness can also identify a high proportion of other chromosomal abnormalities and is associated with major defects of the heart and great arteries, and a wide range of skeletal dysplasias and genetic syndromes. Possible mechanisms for increased nuchal translucency include cardiac failure, venous congestion in the head and neck due to superior mediastinal compression, altered composition of the extracellular matrix, abnormal or delayed development of the lymphatic system, failure of lymphatic drainage due to impaired fetal movements, fetal anemia or congenital infection.

Other benefits of the 11–14-week scan include confirmation that the fetus is alive, accurate dating of the pregnancy, early diagnosis of major fetal defects, and the detection of multiple pregnancies. The early scan also provides reliable identification of chorionicity, which is the main determinant of outcome in multiple pregnancies.

As with the introduction of any new technology into routine clinical practice, it is essential that those undertaking the 11–14-week scan are adequately trained and their results are subjected to rigorous audit. The Fetal Medicine Foundation, under the auspices of the International Society of Ultrasound in Obstetrics and Gynecology, has introduced a process of training and certification to help to establish high standards of scanning on an international basis. The Certificate of Competence in the 11–14-week scan is awarded to those sonographers that can perform the scan to a high standard and can demonstrate a good knowledge of the diagnostic features and management of the conditions identified by this scan.

1

Nuchal translucency and chromosomal defects

'The hair is not black, as in the real Mongol, but of a brownish colour, straight and scanty. The face is flat and broad, and destitute of prominence. The cheeks are roundish, and extended laterally. The eyes are obliquely placed, and the internal canthi more than normally distant from one another. The palpebral fissure is very narrow. The forehead is wrinkled transversely from the constant assistance which the levatores palpebrarum derive from the occipito-frontalis muscle in opening of the eyes. The lips are large and thick with transverse fissures. The tongue is long, thick, and is much roughened. The nose is small. *The skin* has a slight dirty yellowish tinge, and *is deficient in elasticity, giving the appearance of being too large for the body.'*

The above is an extract from the paper 'Observations on an ethnic classification of idiots' by Langdon Down, published in 1866[1]. Down, who was a physician at the London Hospital, coined the phrase Mongolian idiots because he felt that a subgroup of his patients had a resemblance to the Mongolian peoples and this fitted in with his theory of 'retrogression' of ethnic type. Down's theory of ethnic regression was in keeping with Darwin's contemporary scientific reasoning for evolution. In 1924, Crookshank suggested that the regression was not merely to a primitive Oriental human type but also to the orangutan[2]. Even though the theory of ethnic regression was proven to be inaccurate, Down's description of the appearance of the skin was the basis for the observation, made more than one century later, that affected individuals during the 3rd month of intrauterine life, have a subcutaneous collection of fluid behind the neck (Figure 1), which can be visualized by ultrasound as nuchal translucency (Figure 2).

Langdon Down in 1866 and Fraser and Mitchell in 1876 recognized that the condition was congenital, dating from intrauterine life, and in 1914 Goddard found that there was no increased incidence within families[1,3,4]. A number of conditions were

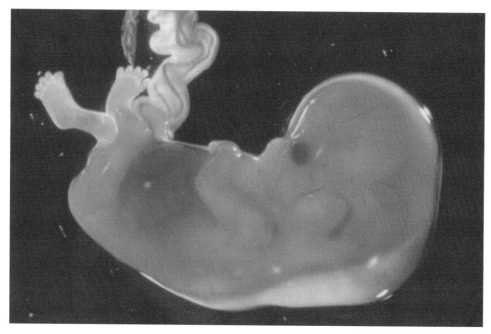

Figure 1 Fetus with subcutaneous collection of fluid at the back of the neck. Image kindly provided by Dr Eva Pajkrt, University of Amsterdam

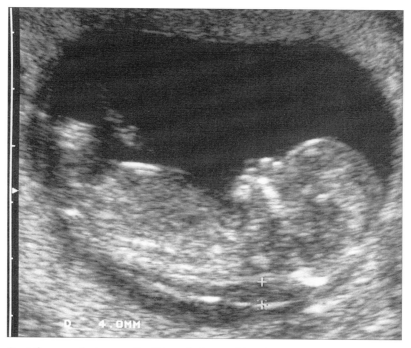

Figure 2 Ultrasound picture of a 12-week fetus with trisomy 21, demonstrating increased nuchal translucency thickness

advocated as potential causes of Down's syndrome, including syphilis, tuberculosis, parental alcoholism, epilepsy, insanity, nervous instability and mental retardation in a close relative, thyroid deficiency, hypoplasia of the fetal adrenal glands, dysfunction of the fetal pituitary and abnormality of the fetal thymus[1,6–13].

The association between Down's syndrome and increased maternal age was noted in 1909 by Shuttleworth[6], who examined 350 cases and reported that:

> 'It would seem fair inference... that more than half of the Mongolian imbeciles in institutions are last-born children, mostly of long families, and that in a considerable proportion – from one-half to *one-third* – *the mothers were at the time of gestation approaching the climacteric period*, and that in consequence the reproductive powers were at a low ebb. Which of the two factors – the advanced age of the mother or her exhaustion by a long series of previous pregnancies – is the more potent factor is open to doubt.'[6]

As a result of the above observation, hypotheses were based upon theoretical degeneration of the ovum[14–16]. However, advanced maternal age could not be the only factor, because, in some cases, there appeared to be a hereditary factor as well. For instance, dizygotic twins were unequally affected whereas monozygotic twins were equally affected[17]. It was also noticed that the condition could be transmitted from mother to baby, and, when more than one member of a family was affected, the dependence on the mother's age was weakened[18–21]. The concept of non-dysjunction in Down's syndrome was suggested by Waardenburg in 1932[22]. In 1934, Bleyer proposed that an unequal migration of chromosomes during cell division may result in trisomy[16].

In 1956, Tjio and Levan, working with improved techniques on cultures of lung fibroblasts, established that the normal diploid chromosome number is 46[23]. In the same year, Ford and Hamerton found that the haploid number was 23 in human spermatocytes[24]. These discoveries led a number of laboratories to study the karyotype in various pathological conditions and in 1959 Lejeune *et al.* and Jacobs *et al.* demonstrated that an extra acrocentric chromosome was present in persons with Down's syndrome, resulting in an aneuploid chromosome number of 47[25,26].

There were familial cases of Down's syndrome which were not the result of trisomy. In 1960 Polani *et al.* examined the chromosomes of a child with Down's syndrome from a 21-year-old mother, there were 46 chromosomes with a centric fusion of two chromosomes (15 : 21)[27]. Familial transmission of this type of translocation was demonstrated by Penrose *et al.* in 1960 in a family with two Down's syndrome sibs[28]. In 1961, Clarke *et al.* reported on a 2-year-old girl with normal intelligence but some physical features suggestive of Down's syndrome; she was discovered to be a mosaic for normal and trisomic cells[29].

Today we know that Down's syndrome occurs when either the whole or a segment of the long arm of chromosome 21 is present in three copies instead of two. This can occur as a result of three separate mechanisms: non-dysjunction, found in about 95% of cases, translocation and mosaicism. In 1991, Antonarakis *et al.* examined DNA polymorphisms in Down's syndrome infants and demonstrated that 95% of non-dysjunction trisomy 21 is maternal in origin[30]. The region that codes for most of the Down's syndrome phenotype is the distal portion of band q21.1 and bands q22.2 and q22.3. This region determines the facial features, heart defects, mental retardation and probably the dermatoglyphic changes in affected individuals[31].

In 1966, 100 years after the original essay of Langdon Down, it became possible to diagnose trisomy 21 prenatally by karyotyping of cultured amniotic fluid cells[32,33].

The first method of screening for trisomy 21, introduced in the early 1970s, was based on the observation of Shuttleworth on the association with advanced maternal age[6]. It was apparent that amniocentesis carried a risk of miscarriage and this in conjunction with the cost implications, meant that prenatal diagnosis could not be offered to the entire pregnant population. Consequently, amniocentesis was initially offered only to women with a minimum age of 40 years. Gradually, as the application of amniocentesis became more widespread and it appeared to be 'safe', the 'high-risk' group was redefined to include women with a minimum age of 35 years; this 'high-risk' group constituted 5% of the pregnant population.

In the last 20 years, two dogmatic policies have emerged in terms of screening. The first, mainly observed in countries with private healthcare systems, adhered to the dogma of the 35 years of age or equivalent risk; since the maternal age of pregnant women has increased in most developed countries, the screen-positive group now constitute about 10% of pregnancies. The second policy, instituted in countries with national health systems, has adhered to the dogma of offering invasive testing to the 5% group of women with the highest risk; in the last 20 years, the cut-off age for invasive testing has therefore increased from 35 to 37 years. In screening by maternal age with a cut-off age of 37 years, 5% of the population are classified as 'high risk' and this group contains about 30% of trisomy 21 babies.

In the late 1980s, a new method of screening was introduced that takes into account not only maternal age but also the concentration of various fetoplacental products in the maternal circulation. At 16 weeks of gestation the median maternal serum concentrations of α-fetoprotein, estriol and human chorionic gonadotropin (hCG) (total and free-β) in trisomy 21 pregnancies are sufficiently different from normal to allow the use of combinations of some or all of these substances to select a 'high-risk' group. This method of screening is more effective than maternal age alone and, for the same rate of invasive testing (about 5%), it can identify about 60% of the fetuses with trisomy 21.

In the 1990s, screening by a combination of maternal age and fetal nuchal translucency thickness at 11–14 weeks of gestation was introduced. This method has now been shown to identify about 75% of affected fetuses for a screen–positive rate of about 5%.

Recent evidence suggests that maternal age can be combined with fetal nuchal translucency and maternal serum biochemistry (free β-hCG and pregnancy-associated plasma protein (PAPP-A)) at 11–14 weeks to identify about 90% of affected fetuses. Furthermore, the development of new methods of biochemical testing, within 30 min of taking a blood sample, has now made it possible to introduce One-Stop Clinics for Assessment of Risk (Figure 3).

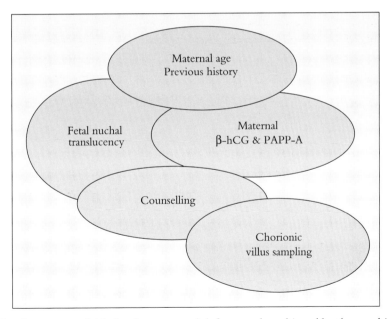

Figure 3 Assessment of risk for chromosomal defects can be achieved by the combination of maternal age and history of previously affected pregnancies, ultrasound measurement of fetal nuchal translucency and biochemical measurement of maternal serum free β-hCG and PAPP-A in an OSCAR at 11–14 weeks of gestation. After counselling, the patient can decide if she wants fetal karyotyping, which can be carried out by chorionic villus sampling in the same visit

CALCULATION OF RISK FOR CHROMOSOMAL DEFECTS

Every woman has a risk that her fetus/baby has a chromosomal defect. In order to calculate the individual risk, it is necessary to take into account the *background risk* (which depends on maternal age, gestation and previous history of chromosomal defects) and multiply this by a series of *factors*, which depend on the results of a series of screening tests carried out during the course of the pregnancy. Every time a test is carried out the *background risk is multiplied by the test factor* to calculate a new risk, which then becomes the background risk for the next test[34]. This process is called *sequential screening*. With the introduction of OSCAR, this can all be achieved in one session at about 12 weeks of pregnancy (Figure 3).

Maternal age and gestation

The risk for many of the chromosomal defects increases with maternal age (Figure 4). Additionally, because fetuses with chromosomal defects are more likely to die *in utero* than normal fetuses, the risk decreases with gestational age (Figure 5).

Estimates of the maternal age-related risk for trisomy 21 at birth are based on two surveys with almost complete ascertainment of the affected patients; in a survey in South Belgium, every neonate was examined for features of trisomy 21 and, in a survey in Sweden, information was verified using several sources such as hospital notes, cytogenetic laboratories, genetic clinics and schools for the mentally handicapped[35,36]. The data from these surveys were used to calculate maternal age-specific incidences of trisomy 21 at birth[37].

During the last decade, with the introduction of maternal serum biochemistry and ultrasound screening for chromosomal defects at different stages of pregnancy, it has become necessary to establish maternal age and gestational age-specific risks for chromosomal defects. Such estimates were derived by comparing the birth prevalence of trisomy 21[37] to the prevalence in women undergoing second-trimester amniocentesis or first-trimester chorionic villus sampling. Rates of spontaneous fetal death between different gestations and delivery at 40 weeks were estimated on the basis of both the observed prevalence in pregnancies that had antenatal fetal karyotyping and the reported prevalence in live births.

Snijders *et al.* examined the prevalence of trisomy 21 in 57 614 women who had fetal karyotyping at 9–16 weeks of gestation for the sole indication of maternal age of 35 years or more; this group included 538 pregnancies with trisomy 21[38–40]. They found that the prevalence of trisomy 21 was higher in early pregnancy than in live births

8

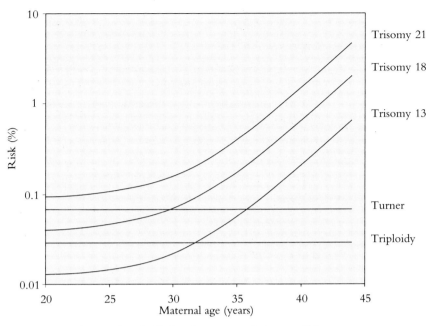

Figure 4 Maternal age-related risk for chromosomal abnormalities

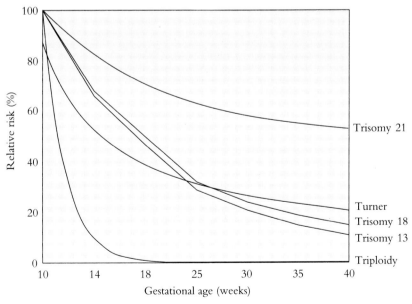

Figure 5 Gestational age-related risk for chromosomal abnormalities. The lines represent the relative risk according to the risk at 10 weeks of gestation

and the estimated rates of fetal loss were 36% from 10 weeks, 30% from 12 weeks, and 21% from 16 weeks[38]. The estimated maternal age and gestational age-related risks for trisomy 21 are given in Table 1.

In a similar study, Halliday *et al.* compared the prevalence of trisomy 21 in 10 545 women having chorionic villus sampling or amniocentesis to the prevalence in live births from 12 921 women of similar age who did not have fetal karyotyping[41]. Their estimated fetal loss rate between 10 weeks and term was 31% and between 16 weeks and term was 18%. Morris *et al.* examined outcome data from 4148 trisomy 21 pregnancies reported to the National Down Syndrome Cytogenetic Register in the UK with correction for elective terminations. Their study population included 441 cases diagnosed at 11–13 weeks of gestation and 2035 cases diagnosed at 16–18 weeks; they estimated that the loss rates between 12 and 16 weeks and term were 31% and 24%, respectively[42]. These estimates for spontaneous loss between the first trimester and term are lower than the 48% reported by Macintosh *et al.* who compared the prevalence

Table 1   Prevalence of trisomy 21 by maternal age and gestational age[38]

Maternal age (years)	Gestational age (weeks)					
	10	*12*	*14*	*16*	*20*	*40*
20	1/983	1/1068	1/1140	1/1200	1/1295	1/1527
25	1/870	1/946	1/1009	1/1062	1/1147	1/1352
30	1/576	1/626	1/668	1/703	1/759	1/895
31	1/500	1/543	1/580	1/610	1/658	1/776
32	1/424	1/461	1/492	1/518	1/559	1/659
33	1/352	1/383	1/409	1/430	1/464	1/547
34	1/287	1/312	1/333	1/350	1/378	1/446
35	1/229	1/249	1/266	1/280	1/302	1/356
36	1/180	1/196	1/209	1/220	1/238	1/280
37	1/140	1/152	1/163	1/171	1/185	1/218
38	1/108	1/117	1/125	1/131	1/142	1/167
39	1/82	1/89	1/95	1/100	1/108	1/128
40	1/62	1/68	1/72	1/76	1/82	1/97
41	1/47	1/51	1/54	1/57	1/62	1/73
42	1/35	1/38	1/41	1/43	1/46	1/55
43	1/26	1/29	1/30	1/32	1/35	1/41
44	1/20	1/21	1/23	1/24	1/26	1/30
45	1/15	1/16	1/17	1/18	1/19	1/23

of trisomy 21 at chorionic villus sampling and birth; the most likely explanation for this high rate (48%), compared to rates derived in the other reports (31%), is that the study included a substantial proportion of cases in which chorionic villus sampling was performed before 10 weeks of gestation[43].

Similar methods were used to produce estimates of risks for other chromosomal abnormalities[40]. The risk for trisomies 18 and 13 increases with maternal age and decreases with gestation; the rate of intrauterine lethality between 12 weeks and 40 weeks is about 80% (Tables 2 and 3). Turner syndrome is usually due to loss of the paternal X chromosome and, consequently, the frequency of conception of 45,X embryos, unlike that of trisomies, is unrelated to maternal age. The prevalence is about 1 per 1500 at 12 weeks, 1 per 3000 at 20 weeks and 1 per 4000 at 40 weeks. For the other sex chromosome abnormalities (47,XXX, 47,XXY and 47,XYY), there is no significant change with maternal age and since the rate of intrauterine lethality is not higher than in chromosomally normal fetuses the overall prevalence (about 1 per 500) does not decrease with gestation. Polyploidy affects about 2% of recognized conceptions but it is highly lethal and thus very rarely observed in live births; the prevalences at 12 and 20 weeks are about 1 per 2000 and 1 per 250 000, respectively[40].

Creating the model for calculation of the maternal and gestational age-specific risks made it possible to counsel patients presenting at different stages of pregnancy about the risk for their fetus having a chromosomal defect and the chance that the pregnancy will result in a live birth with a specific condition. Furthermore, these data can be applied in the evaluation of new ultrasonographic or biochemical methods of screening by calculating the expected prevalence of chromosomal defects in any study group.

Previous affected pregnancy

The risk for trisomies in women who have had a previous fetus or child with a trisomy is higher than the one expected on the basis of their age alone. In a study of 2054 women who had a previous pregnancy with trisomy 21, the risk of recurrence in the subsequent pregnancy was 0.75% higher than the maternal and gestational age-related risk for trisomy 21 at the time of testing. In 750 women who had a previous pregnancy with trisomy 18, the risk of recurrence in the subsequent pregnancy was also about 0.75% higher than the maternal and gestational age-related risk for trisomy 18; the risk for trisomy 21 was not increased[44]. Thus, for a woman aged 35 years who has had a previous baby with trisomy 21, the risk at 12 weeks of gestation increases from 1 in 249 (0.40%) to 1 in 87 (1.15%), and, for a woman aged 25 years, it increases from 1 in 946 (0.106%) to 1 in 117 (0.856%).

Table 2 Risk for trisomy 18 in relation to maternal age and gestation[40]

Maternal age (years)	Gestational age (weeks)					
	10	12	14	16	20	40
20	1/1993	1/2484	1/3015	1/3590	1/4897	1/18013
25	1/1765	1/2200	1/2670	1/3179	1/4336	1/15951
30	1/1168	1/1456	1/1766	1/2103	1/2869	1/10554
31	1/1014	1/1263	1/1533	1/1825	1/2490	1/9160
32	1/860	1/1072	1/1301	1/1549	1/2114	1/7775
33	1/715	1/891	1/1081	1/1287	1/1755	1/6458
34	1/582	1/725	1/880	1/1047	1/1429	1/5256
35	1/465	1/580	1/703	1/837	1/1142	1/4202
36	1/366	1/456	1/553	1/659	1/899	1/3307
37	1/284	1/354	1/430	1/512	1/698	1/2569
38	1/218	1/272	1/330	1/393	1/537	1/1974
39	1/167	1/208	1/252	1/300	1/409	1/1505
40	1/126	1/157	1/191	1/227	1/310	1/1139
41	1/95	1/118	1/144	1/171	1/233	1/858
42	1/71	1/89	1/108	1/128	1/175	1/644

Table 3 Risk of trisomy 13 in relation to maternal age and gestation[40]

Maternal age (years)	Gestational age (weeks)					
	10	12	14	16	20	40
20	1/6347	1/7826	1/9389	1/11042	1/14656	1/42423
25	1/5621	1/6930	1/8314	1/9778	1/12978	1/37567
30	1/3719	1/4585	1/5501	1/6470	1/8587	1/24856
31	1/3228	1/3980	1/4774	1/5615	1/7453	1/21573
32	1/2740	1/3378	1/4052	1/4766	1/6326	1/18311
33	1/2275	1/2806	1/3366	1/3959	1/5254	1/15209
34	1/1852	1/2284	1/2740	1/3222	1/4277	1/12380
35	1/1481	1/1826	1/2190	1/2576	1/3419	1/9876
36	1/1165	1/1437	1/1724	1/2027	1/2691	1/7788
37	1/905	1/1116	1/1339	1/1575	1/2090	1/6050
38	1/696	1/858	1/1029	1/1210	1/1606	1/4650
39	1/530	1/654	1/784	1/922	1/1224	1/3544
40	1/401	1/495	1/594	1/698	1/927	1/2683
41	1/302	1/373	1/447	1/526	1/698	1/2020
42	1/227	1/280	1/335	1/395	1/524	1/1516

The possible mechanism for this increased risk is that a small proportion (less than 5%) of couples with a previously affected pregnancy have parental mosaicism or a genetic defect that interferes with the normal process of dysjunction, so in this group the risk of recurrence is increased substantially. In the majority of couples (more than 95%), the risk of recurrence is not actually increased. Currently available evidence suggests that recurrence is chromosome-specific and, therefore, in the majority of cases, the likely mechanism is parental mosaicism.

Fetal nuchal translucency at the 11–14-week scan

The nuchal translucency normally increases with gestation (crown–rump length). In a fetus with a given crown–rump length, every nuchal translucency measurement represents a factor which is multiplied by the background risk to calculate a new risk. The larger the nuchal translucency, the higher the multiplying factor becomes and therefore the higher the new risk. In contrast, the smaller the nuchal translucency measurement, the smaller the multiplying factor becomes and therefore the lower the new risk (Figure 6).

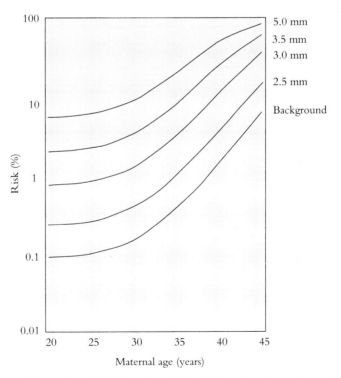

Figure 6 Maternal age-related risk for trisomy 21 at 12 weeks of gestation and the effect of fetal nuchal translucency thickness (NT)

To calculate the multiplying factor (likelihood ratio), it is first necessary to determine the distributions of nuchal translucency thickness in the chromosomally normal and trisomy 21 groups. For a given nuchal translucency, a likelihood ratio is calculated by dividing the percentage of trisomy 21 fetuses by the percentage of normal fetuses with that translucency. The combined risk is then calculated by multiplying the background maternal and gestational age-related risk by the likelihood ratio.

Maternal serum biochemistry at 11–14 weeks

The level of free β-hCG in maternal blood normally decreases with gestation. The higher the β-hCG, the higher the risk for trisomy 21. Again, for a given gestation, each hCG level represents a factor that is multiplied by the background risk to calculate the new risk (Figure 7). The level of PAPP-A in maternal blood normally increases with gestation. The lower the PAPP-A, the higher the risk for trisomy 21. Again, for a given gestation, each PAPP-A level represents a factor that is multiplied by the background risk to calculate the new risk (Figure 7).

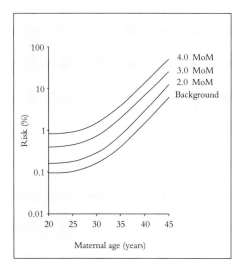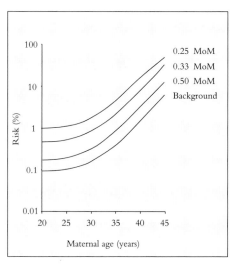

Figure 7 Maternal age-related risk for trisomy 21 at 12 weeks of gestation and the effect of maternal serum free β-hCG (left) and PAPP-A (right)

NUCHAL TRANSLUCENCY THICKNESS

During the second and third trimesters of pregnancy, abnormal accumulation of fluid behind the fetal neck can be classified as nuchal cystic hygroma or nuchal edema. In about 75% of fetuses with cystic hygromas, there is a chromosomal abnormality and, in about 95% of cases, the abnormality is Turner syndrome[45]. Nuchal edema has a diverse etiology; chromosomal abnormalities are found in about one-third of the fetuses and, in about 75% of cases, the abnormality is trisomy 21 or 18. Edema is also associated with fetal cardiovascular and pulmonary defects, skeletal dysplasias, congenital infection and metabolic and hematological disorders; consequently, the prognosis for chromosomally normal fetuses with nuchal edema is poor[46].

In the first trimester, the term translucency is used, because this is the ultrasonographic feature that is observed; during the second trimester, the translucency usually resolves and, in a few cases, it evolves into either nuchal edema or cystic hygromas with or without generalized hydrops.

Measurement of nuchal translucency

Nuchal translucency can be measured successfully by transabdominal ultrasound examination in about 95% of cases; in the others, it is necessary to perform transvaginal sonography. The equipment must be of good quality (about £30 000–50 000), it should have a video-loop function and the callipers should be able to provide measurements to one decimal point. The average time allocated for each fetal scan should be at least 10 minutes. All sonographers performing fetal scans should be capable of reliably measuring the crown–rump length and obtaining a proper sagittal view of the fetal spine. For such sonographers, it is easy to acquire, within a few hours, the skill to measure nuchal translucency thickness. Furthermore, it is essential that the same criteria are used to achieve uniformity of results among different operators (Figure 8):

(1) The minimum fetal crown–rump length should be 45 mm and the maximum 84 mm. The optimal gestational age for measurement of fetal nuchal translucency is 11 to 13[+6] weeks. The success rate for taking a measurement at this gestation is 98–100%, falling to 90% at 14 weeks; from 14 weeks onwards, the fetal position (vertical) makes it more difficult to obtain measurements[47].

(2) The results from transabdominal and transvaginal scanning are similar but reproducibility may be better with the transvaginal method[48].

(3) A good sagittal section of the fetus, as for measurement of fetal crown–rump length, should be obtained.

(4) The magnification should be such that the fetus occupies at least three-quarters of the image. Essentially, the magnification should be increased so that each

increment in the distance between callipers should be only 0.1 mm. A study, in which rat heart ventricles were measured initially by ultrasound and then by dissection, has demonstrated that ultrasound measurements can be accurate to the nearest 0.1–0.2 mm[49].

(5) Care must be taken to distinguish between fetal skin and amnion because, at this gestation, both structures appear as thin membranes. This is achieved by waiting for spontaneous fetal movement away from the amniotic membrane; alternatively, the fetus is bounced off the amnion by asking the mother to cough and/or by tapping the maternal abdomen.

(6) The maximum thickness of the subcutaneous translucency between the skin and the soft tissue overlying the cervical spine should be measured by placing the callipers on the lines as shown in Figure 8. During the scan, more than one measurement must be taken and the maximum one should be recorded.

(7) The nuchal translucency should be measured with the fetus in the neutral position. When the fetal neck is hyperextended the measurement can be increased by 0.6 mm and when the neck is flexed, the measurement can be decreased by 0.4 mm[50].

(8) The umbilical cord may be round the fetal neck in 5–10% of cases and this finding may produce a falsely increased nuchal translucency, adding about 0.8 mm to the measurement[51]. In such cases, the measurements of nuchal translucency above and below the cord are different and, in the calculation of risk, it is more appropriate to use the smaller measurement.

The distribution of nuchal translucency measurements as well as the quality of the images in terms of magnification, section (sagittal or oblique), calliper placement, skin line (nuchal only or nuchal and back) and visualization of the amnion separate from the nuchal membrane are taken into account in the audit of results[52].

The ability to measure nuchal translucency and obtain reproducible results improves with training; good results are achieved after 80 and 100 scans for the transabdominal and the transvaginal routes, respectively[53].

The ability to achieve a reliable measurement of nuchal translucency is dependent on the motivation of the sonographer. A study comparing the results obtained from hospitals where nuchal translucency was used in clinical practice (interventional) compared to those from hospitals where they merely recorded the measurements but

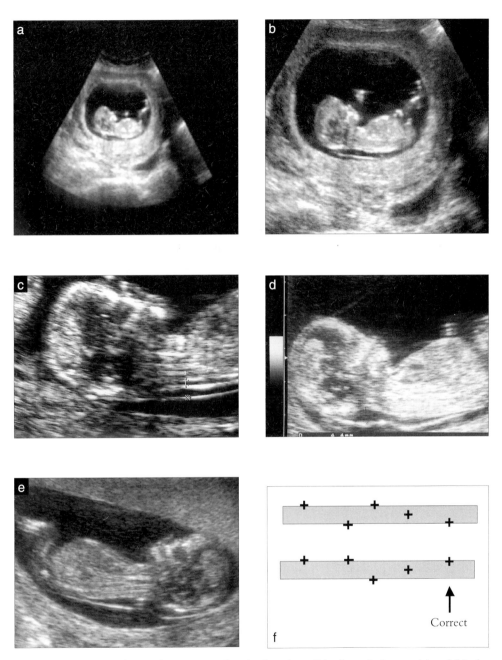

Figure 8 In all the figures there is a good sagittal section of the fetus. In images (a) and (b), the magnification is too small for accurate measurements. The correct magnification is shown in images (c) and (d), where the fetuses are in the neutral position and the amniotic membrane can be clearly seen separated from the nuchal membrane. In image (e), the umbilical cord is round the neck, producing an indentation in the nuchal membrane and the translucency that is larger above than below the cord. The correct placement of the callipers is indicated in diagram (f)

did not act on the results (observational), reported that, in the interventional group, successful measurement of nuchal translucency was achieved in 100% of cases and the measurement was > 2.5 mm in 2.3% of cases; the respective percentages in the observational group were 85% and 12%[54,55].

Appropriate training, high motivation and adherence to a standard technique for the measurement of nuchal translucency are essential prerequisites for good clinical practice. Monni et al. reported that, after modifying their technique of measuring nuchal translucency thickness, by following the guidelines established by The Fetal Medicine Foundation, their detection rate of trisomy 21 improved from 30% to 84%[56].

Repeatability in the measurement of nuchal translucency

A potential criticism of screening by ultrasound is that scanning not only requires highly skilled operators but it is also prone to operator variability. This issue was addressed by a prospective study at 10–14 weeks of gestation in which the nuchal translucency was measured by two of four operators in 200 pregnant women[57]. This study demonstrated that, after an initial measurement, the second one made by the same (intra-) observer or another (inter-) observer varies from the first by less than 0.54 mm and 0.62 mm, respectively in 95% of the cases. Additionally, the study demonstrated that the calliper placement repeatability was similar to the intra-observer and inter-observer repeatabilities, suggesting that a large part of the variation in measurements can be accounted for by the placement of the callipers rather than the generation of the image[57]. Subsequent studies have reported that the intra-observer and inter-observer differences in measurements were less than 0.5 mm in 95% of cases[58,59].

Digital image processing and automation of calliper placement may reduce the variation of measurements[60]. In the meantime, it is best to rely on the mean of two good measurements for the calculation of risk, rather than on a single one.

Increase in nuchal translucency with gestational age

Fetal nuchal translucency thickness increases with crown–rump length[49,61], and therefore it is essential to take gestation into account when determining whether a given translucency thickness is increased. In a study involving more than 100 000 pregnancies, the median increased from 1.2 mm at 11 weeks to 1.9 mm at 13[+6] weeks[62]. Figure 9 illustrates the increases in the 5th, 25th, 50th, 75th and 95th centiles of nuchal translucency with crown–rump length; the 99th centile is about 3.5 mm throughout this gestational range.

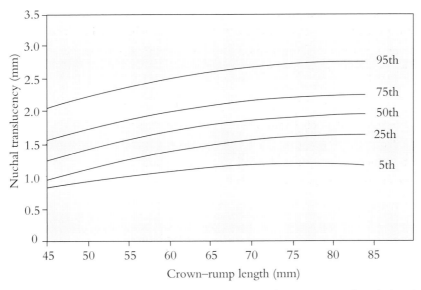

Figure 9 Reference range of fetal nuchal translucency with crown–rump length showing the 5th, 25th, 50th, 75th and 95th centiles

Observational studies: increased nuchal translucency and chromosomal defects

In the early 1990s, several reports of small series in high-risk pregnancies demonstrated a possible association between increased nuchal translucency and chromosomal defects in the first trimester of pregnancy (Table 4)[63–80]. Although the mean prevalence of chromosomal defects in 20 series involving a total of 1698 patients was 29%, there were large differences between the studies with the prevalence ranging from 11% to 88%. This variation in results presumably reflects differences in the maternal age distributions of the populations examined as well as in the definition of the minimum abnormal translucency thickness, which ranged from 2 mm to 10 mm.

Subsequently, a series of screening studies in high-risk pregnancies were carried out; these involved measurement of nuchal translucency thickness immediately before fetal karyotyping, mainly for advanced maternal age. Pandya *et al.* examined a total of 1273 pregnancies and reported that the nuchal translucency thickness was above the 95th centile of the normal range in about 80% of trisomy 21 fetuses[81]. Similar findings were obtained in an additional four studies of pregnancies undergoing first-trimester fetal karyotyping[73,74,76,78]. However, in another study involving 1819 pregnancies, nuchal translucency thickness of ≥ 3 mm identified only 30% of the chromosomally abnormal fetuses (no data were provided specifically for trisomy 21) and the false-positive rate was 3.2%[72].

An important finding of the screening studies in high-risk pregnancies was that the prevalence of chromosomal defects is dependent on both fetal nuchal translucency thickness and maternal age. For example, in a study of 1015 pregnancies with increased fetal nuchal translucency thickness at 10–14 weeks of gestation, the observed numbers of trisomies 21, 18 and 13 in fetuses with translucencies of 3 mm, 4 mm, 5 mm and > 6 mm were approximately 3 times, 18 times, 28 times and 36 times higher than the respective number expected on the basis of maternal age[67]. The incidences of Turner syndrome and triploidy were 9 times and 8 times higher, whilst the incidence of other sex chromosome aneuploidies was similar to that expected[67].

Table 4 Summary of reported series on first-trimester fetal nuchal translucency (NT) providing data on gestational age (GA) in weeks, criteria for diagnosis of increased NT thickness and the presence of associated chromosomal defects

Author	GA (weeks)	NT (mm)	n	Abnormal karyotype					
				Total	T21	T18	T13	45,X	Other
Johnson 1993[63]	10–14	≥2.0	68	41 (60%)	16	9	2	9	5
Hewitt 1993[64]	10–14	≥2.0	29	12 (41%)	5	3	1	2	1
Shulman 1992[65]	10–13	≥2.5	32	15 (47%)	4	4	3	4	—
Nicolaides 1992[66]	10–13	≥3.0	88	33 (38%)	21	8	2	—	2
Pandya 1995[67]	10–13	≥3.0	1015	194 (19%)	101	51	13	14	15
Szabo & Gellen 1990[68]	11–12	≥3.0	8	7 (88%)	7	—	—	—	—
Wilson et al. 1992[69]	8–11	≥3.0	14	3 (21%)	—	—	—	1	2
Ville et al. 1992[70]	9–14	≥3.0	29	8 (28%)	4	3	1	—	—
Trauffer et al. 1994[71]	10–14	≥3.0	43	21 (49%)	9	4	1	4	3
Brambati et al. 1995[72]	8–15	≥3.0	70	8 (11%)	?	?	?	?	?
Comas et al. 1995[73]	9–13	≥3.0	51	9 (18%)	4	4	—	—	1
Szabo et al. 1995[74]	9–12	≥3.0	96	43 (45%)	28	10	—	2	3
Nadel et al. 1993[75]	10–15	≥4.0	63	43 (68%)	15	15	1	10	2
Savoldelli et al. 1993[76]	9–12	≥4.0	24	19 (79%)	15	2	1.	1	—
Schulte-Vallentin 1992[77]	10–14	≥4.0	8	7 (88%)	7	—	—	—	—
van Zalen-Sprock 1992[78]	10–14	≥4.0	18	6 (28%)	3	1	—	1	1
Cullen 1990[79]	11–13	≥6.0	29	15 (52%)	6	2	—	4	3
Suchet 1992[80]	8–14	≥10.0	13	8 (62%)	—	—	—	7	1
Total	8–15	2–10	1698	492 (29%)	245	116	25	59	39

T21, trisomy 21; T18, trisomy 18; T13, trisomy 13

Implementation of nuchal translucency screening in routine practice

There are nine studies that have examined the implementation of nuchal translucency screening in routine practice and the results are summarized in Table 5[54,74,82–88]. The number of trisomy 21 pregnancies in all but one[86] of these studies is too small to allow assessment of the sensitivity of the test. However, these studies demonstrate a series of important points:

(1) It is possible to measure nuchal translucency successfully during a routine first-trimester scan in 96–100% of cases, provided that, first, the gestation is 11–14 weeks and, second, the sonographers are motivated to take such a measurement. Thus, in the two studies that examined the feasibility of measuring nuchal translucency but in which (a) they included patients from as early as 8 weeks, and (b) no action was taken on the results of the translucency measurement, such a measurement was obtained in only 58% and 66% of cases, respectively[83,84].

(2) The false-positive rate varied from as low as 0.8[86] to as high as 6.3%[54,84], demonstrating the need for unifying the criteria in (a) obtaining the appropriate image, (b) calliper placement, and (c) using the same normal range and same cut-off.

Table 5 Studies examining the implementation of fetal nuchal translucency (NT) screening

Author	Gestation (weeks)	n	Successful measurement	NT cut-off (mm)	FPR	DR trisomy 21
Pandya et al. 1995[82]	10–14	1 763	100%	> 2.5	3.6%	3 of 4 (75%)
Szabo et al. 1995[74]	9–12	3 380	100%	> 3.0	1.6%	28 of 31 (90%)
Bewley et al. 1995[83]	8–13	1 704	66%	> 3.0	6.0%	1 of 3 (33%)
Bower et al. 1995[54]	8–14	1 481	97%	> 3.0	6.3%	4 of 8 (50%)
Kornman et al. 1996[84]	8–13	923	58%	> 3.0	6.3%	2 of 4 (50%)
Zimmerman et al. 1996[85]	10–13	1 131	100%	> 3.0	1.9%	2 of 3 (67%)
Taipale et al. 1997[86]	10–16	10 010	99%	> 3.0	0.8%	7 of 13 (54%)
Hafner et al. 1998[87]	10–14	4 371	100%	> 2.5	1.7%	4 of 7 (57%)
Pajkrt et al. 1998[88]	10–14	1 547	96%	> 3.0	2.2%	6 of 9 (67%)

FPR, false-positive rate; DR, detection rate

The Frimley Park Hospital, Camberley and St. Peter's Hospital, Chertsey, UK[82] Frimley Park and St. Peter's are general hospitals within the NHS offering routine antenatal care, and their combined annual number of deliveries is approximately 6000. Prior to the introduction of nuchal translucency scanning, the policy of these hospitals was to offer amniocentesis to women aged 35 years or older. During 1993 there were 11 fetuses with Down's syndrome and only two of these were detected prenatally. Subsequently, nuchal translucency screening at 10–14 weeks of gestation was introduced and the implementation of this policy was achieved without the need for increasing the number of staff or the equipment. Women with fetal translucency of 2.5 mm or more were offered fetal karyotyping. In addition women aged 35 years or older were offered amniocentesis at 16 weeks' gestation. The data of the first 5 months after the introduction of the new policy were analyzed following completion of the pregnancies. During this period, 74% of women delivering in the two hospitals attended for first-trimester scanning and the nuchal translucency was successfully measured in all pregnancies. The nuchal translucency was raised in 3.6% of cases and the total percentage of invasive procedures was 5.1%. All four cases of Down's syndrome that occurred in this period were diagnosed prenatally[82].

University College Hospital, London, UK[83]   In a screening study of 1704 women with singleton pregnancies attending University College Hospital, London, for routine antenatal care at 8–14 weeks of gestation, transabdominal ultrasound examination was performed. In 20% of cases, the sonographers forgot to measure the nuchal translucency thickness. In a further 18% of those women in whom a measurement was attempted, this was unsuccessful. In 28% of the 1127 cases in whom measurements were made, the scans were carried out before 10 weeks of gestation. The nuchal translucency was ≥ 3 mm in 6% of the cases. The population contained three fetuses with trisomy 21, all in women aged ≥ 39 years, and increased nuchal translucency was found in one[83].

Queen Charlotte's and Guy's Hospitals, London, UK[54]   This report combined the data from two centers; in one the study was observational and in the other it was interventional. The nuchal translucency was ≥ 3 mm in four (50%) of the eight trisomy 21 pregnancies. In the interventional center, 969 pregnancies were examined, the nuchal translucency was successfully measured in all cases and the translucency was ≥ 3 mm in 20 (2.0%) of the 966 chromosomally normal pregnancies. In contrast, in the observational center, 512 pregnancies were examined, the nuchal translucency was successfully measured in 470 (92%) of cases and the translucency was ≥ 3 mm in 73 (14.5%) of the 505 chromosomally normal pregnancies. These results suggest that the accuracy of measurements depends on the motivation of the sonographers[54].

University Hospital, Groningen, The Netherlands[84]   This was a screening study of an apparently low-risk population, but in 54% of the cases the mothers were ≥ 36 years old or had a history of a previous chromosomally abnormal fetus/child. In total, 923 fetuses were scanned transabdominally at ≤ 13 weeks of gestation by four ultrasonographers who were instructed not to take more than 3 minutes in making a nuchal translucency measurement. In 54% of cases, the fetal crown–rump length was < 33 mm. Furthermore, in 42% of cases, the nuchal translucency could not be measured. In this population, there were seven cases of trisomy 21 and the authors suggested that the sensitivity of nuchal translucency screening is low because only two of the fetuses had increased translucency. However, in reality, only three of the fetuses with trisomy 21 had a crown–rump length of > 38 mm and a nuchal translucency measurement, and in two of these the translucency was increased[84].

Helsinki University Hospital and Jorvi Hospital, Finland[86]   In this study, transvaginal sonography was performed in 10 010 singleton pregnancies at 10–16 weeks of gestation. Scans were performed by one of six sonographers who were successful in obtaining an ultrasound measurement in 98.6% of cases. Increased nuchal translucency (≥ 3 mm) was observed in 76 (0.8%) of the fetuses and this group included seven (54%) of the 13 fetuses with trisomy 21; the sensitivity for pregnancies at 10–14 weeks was 66% (four of six), for a screen-positive rate of only 0.9%[86].

Danube Hospital, Vienna, Austria[87]   In a screening study of 4371 women with singleton pregnancies attending a government hospital in Vienna for routine antenatal care at 10–14 weeks of gestation, transabdominal ultrasound examination was performed and the fetal nuchal translucency thickness was successfully measured in all cases. The nuchal translucency thickness was ≥ 2.5 mm in 1.7% of the cases and this group included three (43%) of seven with trisomy 21[87].

Academic Medical Center, Amsterdam, The Netherlands[88]   This study examined 1547 pregnancies, including 24% aged > 36 years old, at 10–14 weeks. Scans were performed by one of six sonographers who were successful in obtaining an ultrasound measurement in 96% of cases. Nuchal translucency was ≥ 3 mm in 33 (2.2%) cases and this group included six (67%) of the nine fetuses with trisomy 21[88].

Albert Szent-Gyorgyi Medical University Hospital, Szeged, Hungary[74]   In this study involving 3380 women at 9–12 weeks of gestation, nuchal translucency was successfully measured transvaginally in all cases. Increased translucency (≥ 3 mm) was observed in 81 (2.4%) of fetuses and this group included 28 (90%) of 31 fetuses with trisomy 21[74].

University Hospital, Zurich, Switzerland[85]   In this study, nuchal translucency was measured in 1131 pregnancies at 10–13 weeks of gestation. Increased translucency (≥ 3 mm) was observed in 24 (2.1%) of fetuses and this group included two (67%) of three fetuses with trisomy 21[85].

Screening by a combination of maternal age and fetal nuchal translucency

The Multicenter Screening Study

In a multicenter study in the UK, involving the Harris Birthright Centre and four District General Hospitals (St. Peters, Chertsey; Frimley Park, Camberly; Queen Mary's, Sidcup; Heatherwood, Ascot), nuchal translucency screening at 10–14 weeks of gestation was carried out in 20 804 pregnancies, including 164 cases of chromosomal abnormalities[61]. This study demonstrated that:

(1) In normal pregnancies, nuchal translucency thickness increases with gestation;

(2) In chromosomally abnormal pregnancies, nuchal translucency is increased;

(3) The risk for trisomies can be derived by multiplying the background maternal age and gestation-related risk by a likelihood ratio, which depends on the degree of deviation in nuchal translucency measurement from the expected normal median for that crown–rump length;

(4) In about 5% of pregnancies, the estimated risk for trisomy 21 was at least 1 in 100 and this group included 80% of fetuses with trisomy 21 and 77% of those with other chromosomal abnormalities. Because the maternal age of the screened population was higher than in Britain as a whole, it was estimated that the cut-off risk to include 5% of the British population (median maternal age of 28 years) is 1 in 300; using this cut-off, the sensitivity of the test for trisomy 21 was estimated to be about 80%.

The Fetal Medicine Foundation Ongoing Multicenter Project

There are now 43 countries with centers approved by The Fetal Medicine Foundation for carrying out nuchal translucency screening. In the audit of results from the first 100 000 pregnancies examined in the UK, the nuchal translucency was above the 95th centile in more than 70% of fetuses with trisomy 21[62]. The scans were carried out by 306 appropriately trained sonographers in 22 centers. In each pregnancy, the fetal crown–rump length and nuchal translucency were measured and the risk of trisomy 21 was calculated from the maternal age and gestational age-related prevalence, multiplied by a likelihood ratio depending on the deviation in nuchal translucency from normal (Figures 10–12). The distribution of risks was determined and the sensitivity of a cut-off risk of 1 in 300 was calculated[62].

In total, 100 311 singleton pregnancies were examined and follow-up was obtained from 96 127 cases, including 326 with trisomy 21 and 325 with other chromosomal abnormalities. The median gestation at the time of screening was 12 weeks (range 10–14 weeks) and the median maternal age was 31 years (range 14–49 years); in 13 315 (13.3%) cases, the maternal age was at least 37 years. The fetal nuchal translucency was above the 95th centile for crown–rump length in 4210 (4.4%) of the normal pregnancies and in 234 (71.8%) of those with trisomy 21 (Figure 10). The estimated risk for

24

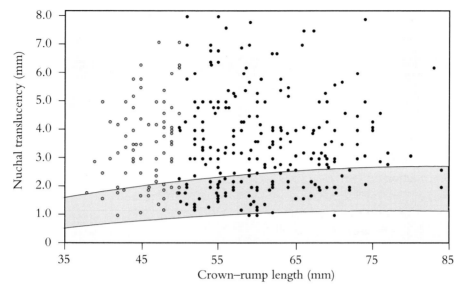

Figure 10 Nuchal translucency measurement in 326 trisomy 21 fetuses plotted on the normal range for crown–rump length (95th and 5th centiles)[62]

trisomy 21 based on maternal age and fetal nuchal translucency was above 1 in 300 in 7907 (8.3%) of the normal pregnancies and in 268 (82.2%) of those with trisomy 21. For a screen-positive rate of 5%, the sensitivity was 77% (95% confidence interval (CI) 72–82%)[62].

Table 6 illustrates the observed prevalence of trisomy 21 according to the predicted risk based on maternal age and fetal nuchal translucency thickness. These results demonstrate the high degree of accuracy of the model.

Table 6 Accuracy of estimated risk (median and range) for trisomy 21 by a combination of maternal age and fetal nuchal translucency thickness[62]

Estimated risk	n	Trisomy 21	Observed prevalence
1 in 7 (1 in 2–1 in 19)	1 305	187	1 in 7
1 in 59 (1 in 20–1 in 99)	2 011	49	1 in 41
1 in 198 (1 in 100–1 in 299)	5 096	32	1 in 159
1 in 632 (1 in 300–1 in 999)	18 279	31	1 in 614
1 in 1504 (1 in 1000–1 in 1999)	19 445	14	1 in 1389
1 in 3702 (1 in 2000–1 in 6000)	49 991	13	1 in 3846

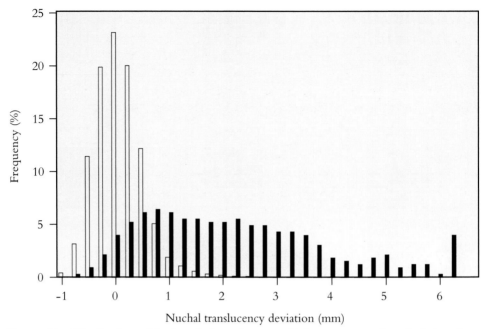

Figure 11 Distribution of fetal nuchal translucency thickness expressed as deviation from expected normal median for crown–rump length in chromosomally normal fetuses (open bars) and 326 with trisomy 21 (solid bars)[62]

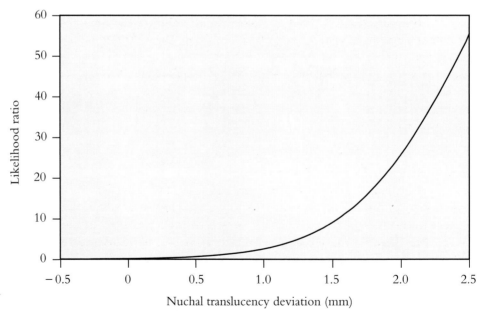

Figure 12 Likelihood ratios for trisomy 21 in relation to the deviation in fetal nuchal translucency thickness from the expected normal median for crown–rump length[62]

Other screening studies using nuchal translucency expressed as centiles

The Royal Free Hospital, London, UK[89]   In this study, nuchal translucency was measured at 11–14 weeks in 2281 pregnancies with a mean maternal age of 30 years. The nuchal translucency was ≥ 99th centile for crown–rump length in six of the eight (75%) fetuses with trisomy 21. In the two trisomic pregnancies with low nuchal translucency, maternal serum biochemistry at 16 weeks also showed a low risk[89].

Homerton–St. Bartholomew's–Royal London Hospitals, London, UK[90]   In   this   study, women were offered screening by a combination of maternal age and fetal nuchal translucency at 12–13 weeks. A risk cut-off of 1 in 100 was used to identify the high-risk group; the screen-positive rate was 2.6% and this group contained five (71%) of seven cases of trisomy 21[90].

The Greek multicenter study[91]   This was a multicenter study involving routine measurement of nuchal translucency thickness in 3550 pregnancies at 10–14 weeks of gestation. The median maternal age was 29 years and 7.8% were aged 37 years or more. All five ultrasonographers had received a Certificate of Competence in first-trimester scanning by The Fetal Medicine Foundation. Successful measurements of nuchal translucency were obtained in all cases. The risk of trisomy 21, based on a combination of maternal age and fetal nuchal translucency thickness, was ≥ 1 in 300 in 4.9% of the population and this high-risk group contained 10 of the 11 (91%) fetuses with trisomy 21, and all five cases of trisomies 18 or 13[91].

Ospedale Regionale per le Microcitemie, Cagliari, Italy[56]   Monni *et al.* introduced screening on the basis of fetal nuchal translucency in January 1995; by May 1995 a total of 1176 patients with a crown–rump length of 17–85 mm had been examined. They identified only 30% of fetuses with a chromosome abnormality using a cut-off of ≥ 3 mm. In 1996, sonographers modified the technique to follow guidelines established by The Fetal Medicine Foundation. In the subsequent year, the detection rate based on maternal age and fetal nuchal translucency thickness improved to 84%[56].

University of Florence Hospital, Florence, Italy[92]   Biagiotti *et al.* evaluated screening on the basis of fetal nuchal translucency in 3241 pregnancies examined at 9–13 weeks of gestation. The authors compared two different methods, delta nuchal translucency and multiples of the expected median. They concluded that expressing values as multiples of the median, as used in screening with maternal serum biochemistry, provides optimal results. Screening based on maternal age and fetal nuchal translucency identified 59% of the cases for a 5% false-positive rate[92].

Cervello Hospital, Palermo, Italy[93]   Orlandi *et al.* evaluated screening for aneuploidy with fetal nuchal translucency and maternal serum biochemistry at 9–14 weeks of gestation. Nuchal translucency was measured in 744 pregnancies and was above the 95th centile in four (57%) of seven fetuses with trisomy 21 and in 42 (5.8%) of the 730 normal fetuses. The findings further indicated that screening by a combination of maternal age, fetal nuchal translucency and maternal serum biochemistry at 9–14 weeks of gestation identifies 87% of affected pregnancies for a 5% false-positive rate[93].

Lethality of trisomy 21 fetuses with increased nuchal translucency

Screening for chromosomal defects in the first rather than the second trimester has the advantage of earlier prenatal diagnosis and consequently less traumatic termination of pregnancy for those couples who choose this option. A potential disadvantage is that earlier screening preferentially identifies those chromosomally abnormal pregnancies that are destined to miscarry. Approximately 30% of affected fetuses die between 12 weeks of gestation and term[38,41,42]. This issue of preferential intrauterine lethality of chromosomal defects is, of course, a potential criticism of all methods of antenatal screening, including second-trimester maternal serum biochemistry; the estimated rate of intrauterine lethality between 16 weeks and term is about 20%[38,41,42]. This section examines the interrelation between increased nuchal translucency in trisomy 21 and fetal lethality.

Decision to continue with the pregnancy after the diagnosis of trisomy 21

In a study of 108 fetuses with trisomy 21 diagnosed in the first trimester because of increased nuchal translucency, the parents chose to continue with the pregnancy in five cases, whereas in 103 cases they opted for termination[94]. Trisomy 21 was also diagnosed in one of the fetuses in a twin pregnancy where the parents elected to avoid invasive prenatal diagnosis or selective fetocide[94]. In five of the six fetuses, the translucency resolved, and at the second-trimester scan the nuchal-fold thickness was normal (less than 7 mm). All six trisomy 21 babies were born alive. One had a major atrioventricular septal defect and died at the age of 6 months. Another two of the babies had small ventricular septal defects and these were managed conservatively, awaiting spontaneous closure. These data suggest that increased nuchal translucency does not necessarily identify those trisomic fetuses that are destined to die *in utero*.

Decision to terminate the pregnancy after the diagnosis of trisomy 21

In a study of 70 pregnancies with trisomy 21 diagnosed at 12 (range 11–14) weeks of gestation, the parents opted for elective termination which was carried out at 14 (12–20) weeks. Ultrasound examination to determine if the fetus was alive was carried out at the time of chorionic villus sampling as well as just before termination[95]. Eight fetuses died in the interval between chorionic villus sampling and termination and the rate of lethality increased with nuchal translucency thickness from 5.3% for those with nuchal translucency of 0–3 mm to 23.5% for nuchal translucency of ≥ 7 mm. Assuming that the relative rate of intrauterine lethality of trisomy 21 fetuses according to the nuchal translucency thickness remains the same throughout pregnancy, it was estimated that a policy of screening by maternal age and fetal nuchal translucency followed by selective termination of affected fetuses would be associated with at least a 70% reduction in the live birth incidence of trisomy 21.

Data from The Fetal Medicine Foundation Multicenter Project

Among the 100 000 pregnancies that were screened within the multicenter project, trisomy 21 was diagnosed, prenatally or at birth, in 326 cases[62]. On the basis of the maternal age distribution in this population and the maternal age-related prevalence of trisomy 21 in live births, it was estimated that 266 babies with trisomy 21 would have been born alive had there not been any antenatal testing and selective termination of affected pregnancies.

In the screen-negative group (estimated risk of less than 1 in 300), there were 35 live births with trisomy 21 and 23 other cases where the pregnancies were terminated following prenatal diagnosis. On the extreme assumption that all 23 of these pregnancies would have resulted in live births, then the number of trisomy 21 live births in the screen-negative group would have been 58, or 22% of the total 266 potential live births with trisomy 21. Consequently, assessment of risk by a combination of maternal age and fetal nuchal translucency, followed by invasive diagnostic testing for those with a risk of ≥ 1 in 300, and selective termination of affected fetuses would have reduced the potential live birth prevalence of trisomy 21 by at least 78% (208 of 266)[62].

INCREASED NUCHAL TRANSLUCENCY AND OTHER CHROMOSOMAL DEFECTS

In The Fetal Medicine Foundation Multicenter Project of screening for trisomy 21 by a combination of maternal age and fetal nuchal translucency thickness at 10–14 weeks, 325 with chromosomal abnormalities other than trisomy 21 were identified[62]. In 229 (70.5%) of these, the fetal nuchal translucency was above the 95th centile of the normal range for crown–rump length (Table 7). Furthermore, in 253 (77.9%) of the pregnancies, the estimated risk for trisomy 21, based on maternal age and fetal nuchal translucency, was more than 1 in 300.

In trisomy 21, the median nuchal translucency thickness is about 2.0 mm above the normal median for crown–rump length. The corresponding values for trisomies

Table 7 Nuchal translucency thickness above the 95th centile and an estimated risk for trisomy 21 of more than 1 in 300 in pregnancies with chromosomal abnormalities other than trisomy 21

Fetal karyotype	n	Nuchal translucency > 95th centile	Estimated risk > 1 in 300
Trisomy 18	119	89 (74.8%)	97 (81.5%)
Trisomy 13	46	33 (71.7%)	37 (80.4%)
Turner syndrome	54	47 (87.0%)	48 (88.9%)
Triploidy	32	19 (59.4%)	20 (62.5%)
Other*	74	41 (55.4%)	51 (79.7%)
Total	325	229 (70.5%)	253 (77.9%)

*Deletions, partial trisomies, unbalanced translocations, sex chromosome aneuploidies

18 and 13, triploidy and Turner syndrome are 4.0 mm, 2.5 mm, 1.5 mm and 7.0 mm, respectively.

In addition to increased nuchal translucency, there are other characteristic sonographic findings in these fetuses (Table 8). In trisomy 18, there is early onset intrauterine growth restriction, relative bradycardia and, in about 30% of the cases, there is an associated exomphalos (Figure 13)[96]. Trisomy 13 is characterized by fetal tachycardia, observed in about two-thirds of the cases, early onset intrauterine growth restriction, and holoprosencephaly or exomphalos in about 30% of the cases[97]. Turner syndrome is characterized by fetal tachycardia, observed in about 50% of the cases, and early onset intrauterine growth restriction[98]. In triploidy, there is early onset asymmetrical intrauterine growth restriction (Figure 14), relative bradycardia, holoprosencephaly, exomphalos or posterior fossa cyst in about 40% of cases and molar changes in the placenta in about one-third of cases[99].

Table 8 Ultrasound findings in chromosomally abnormal fetuses at 10–14 weeks of gestation

Fetal karyotype	Ultrasound findings
Trisomy 18	growth restriction, bradycardia, exomphalos
Trisomy 13	growth restriction, tachycardia, holoprosencephaly, exomphalos
Turner syndrome	growth restriction, tachycardia, large nuchal translucency (cystic hygromas)
Triploidy	growth restriction, bradycardia, holoprosencephaly, posterior fossa cyst, exomphalos, molar placenta

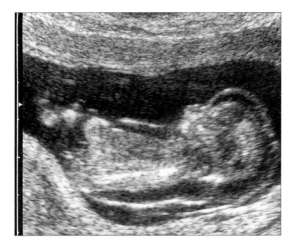

Figure 13 Increased nuchal translucency and exomphalos in a trisomy 18 fetus at 12 weeks of gestation

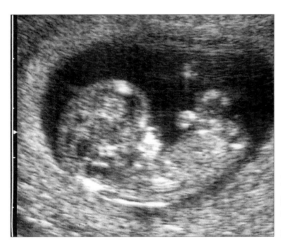

Figure 14 Severe asymmetrical growth restriction in a 13-week fetus with triploidy. The placenta looks normal

CROWN–RUMP LENGTH IN CHROMOSOMALLY ABNORMAL FETUSES

Low birth weight is a common feature of many chromosomal abnormalities[100,101]. Furthermore, prenatal studies during the second and third trimesters of pregnancy have reported a high prevalence of aneuploidies in severe intrauterine growth restriction[102].

Studies examining first-trimester growth in chromosomally abnormal fetuses have demonstrated that trisomy 18 and triploidy are associated with moderately severe growth restriction, trisomy 13 and Turner syndrome with mild growth restriction, whereas in trisomy 21 growth is essentially normal (Tables 9 and 10, Figure 15).

In 10–45% of pregnancies, women are uncertain of their last menstrual period, they have irregular menstrual cycles or they became pregnant soon after stopping the oral contraceptive pill[109,110]. Additionally, because of considerable variations in the day of ovulation, in approximately 10% of women with certain dates and regular 28-day cycles, there is a discrepancy of more than 7 days in gestation calculated from the menstrual history and by ultrasound[111]. For these reasons, accurate dating of pregnancy necessitates ultrasonographic examination. A policy of routine pregnancy dating by measurement of crown–rump length will not affect the interpretation of results in screening by nuchal translucency thickness for trisomy 21. In the case of the other chromosomal defects, dating by crown–rump length will actually improve their detection since nuchal translucency normally increases with gestation.

Table 9 Harris Birthright Research Centre for Fetal Medicine 10–14-week Ultrasound Study. In 787 chromosomally abnormal pregnancies, where the women were certain of their dates and had regular menstrual cycles of 26–30 days, the difference in gestation between that estimated by measurement of fetal crown–rump length and menstrual dates was calculated

Chromosomal defect	n	Growth deficit
Trisomy 21	431	0.7 days
Trisomy 18	169	5.9 days
Trisomy 13	73	3.1 days
Triploidy	30	8.5 days
Turner syndrome	84	1.8 days

Table 10 Studies reporting on first-trimester growth of chromosomally abnormal fetuses

Author	Trisomy 21	Trisomy 18	Trisomy 13	Triploidy	Turner
Lynch & Berkowitz 1989[103]		5*			
Drugan et al. 1992[104]	27†				
Khun et al. 1995[105]	72	32*	11	3	5
Macintosh et al. 1995[106]	14‡				
Bahado-Singh et al. 1997[107]	86	28*	14*	6	8
Jauniaux et al. 1997[99]				18*	
Schemmer et al. 1997[108]	92	49*	19*	8*	8
Sherrod et al. 1997[96]		98*			

*Significantly reduced crown–rump length; †non-significant deficit in crown–rump length by the equivalent of 1 day; ‡non-significant deficit in crown–rump length by the equivalent of 2 days

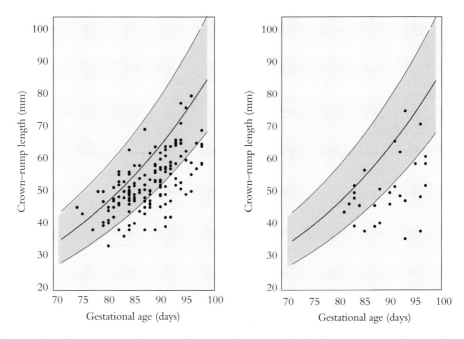

Figure 15 Crown–rump length in fetuses with trisomy 18 (left) and triploidy (right), plotted on the normal range for gestation (mean, 95th and 5th centiles)

FETAL HEART RATE IN CHROMOSOMALLY ABNORMAL FETUSES

Studies examining first-trimester fetal heart rate in chromosomally abnormal fetuses have demonstrated that trisomy 13 and Turner syndrome are associated with tachycardia, whereas in trisomy 18 and triploidy there is a tendency for bradycardia. In trisomy 21, there is a mild increase in fetal heart rate (Table 11, Figure 16).

Table 11 Harris Birthright Research Centre for Fetal Medicine 10–14-week Ultrasound Study. The fetal heart rate in 842 chromosomally abnormal pregnancies is presented as a percentage of cases above the 95th and 50th and below the 5th centiles of the normal range for crown–rump length, derived from 10 083 normal pregnancies

Chromosomal defect	< 5th centile	> 50th centile	> 95th centile
Trisomy 21 ($n = 451$)	27 (6.0%)	256 (56.8%)	62 (13.7%)
Trisomy 18 ($n = 176$)	33 (18.8%)	65 (36.9%)	9 (5.1%)
Trisomy 13 ($n = 77$)	2 (2.6%)	72 (93.5%)	53 (68.8%)
Triploidy ($n = 42$)	15 (35.7%)	13 (31.0%)	2 (4.8%)
Turner syndrome ($n = 96$)	2 (2.1%)	85 (88.5%)	51 (53.1%)

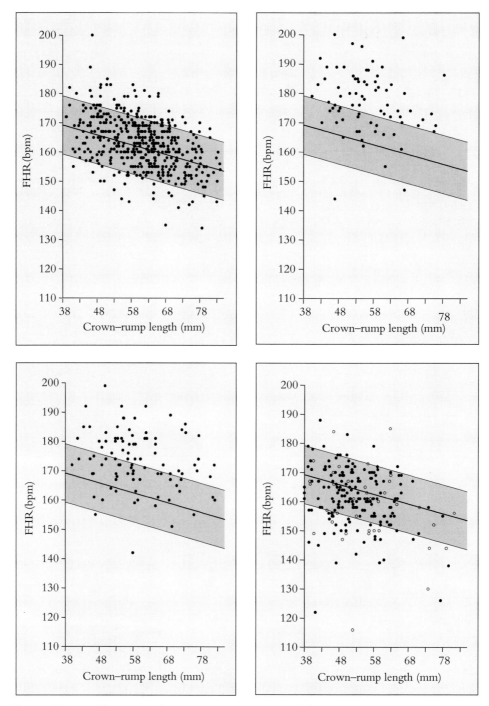

Figure 16 Fetal heart rate (FHR) in trisomy 21 (top left), trisomy 13 (top right), Turner syndrome (bottom left) and triploidy (○) and trisomy 18 (●) (bottom right) plotted on the normal range for gestation (median, 95th and 5th centiles)

In a study of 10 083 normal pregnancies at the Harris Birthright Research Centre for Fetal Medicine, the mean fetal heart rate decreased with gestation from 169 bpm at a fetal crown–rump length of 38 mm to 154 bpm at a crown–rump length of 84 mm. The data were normally distributed and the 95th and 5th centiles were 10 bpm above and below the appropriate normal mean for crown–rump length, respectively. In trisomy 13, Turner syndrome and trisomy 21, the respective mean fetal heart rates were 14 bpm, 11.4 bpm and 1.4 bpm above the normal mean for crown–rump length, whereas, in trisomy 18 and triploidy, the fetal heart rates were 3.4 bpm and 4.8 bpm below the normal mean, respectively.

Previous studies on trisomy 21 fetuses have reported conflicting results. In a longitudinal study of one trisomy 21 fetus at 6–9 weeks of gestation, the heart rate was consistently below the 3rd centile of the normal range[112]. In another cross-sectional study of five affected fetuses at 7–13 weeks, the heart rate was always within the normal range[113]. A study of 17 trisomy 21 fetuses at 10–13 weeks reported that, in 23.5% of cases, the heart rate was either above the 97th centile or below the 2.5th centile[114]. In another study of 85 trisomy 21 fetuses at 10–14 weeks, the heart rate was above the 95th centile in 21% of cases and the increase in heart rate was not related to fetal nuchal translucency thickness. This finding raises the possibility of including fetal heart rate in the model of risk assessment for trisomy 21 along with maternal age and fetal nuchal translucency[115]. In our extended series of 451 fetuses with trisomy 21 at 10–14 weeks, 13.7% had a heart rate above the 95th centile (Table 11).

In normal pregnancy, the fetal heart rate increases from about 110 bpm at 5 weeks of gestation, to 170 bpm at 9 weeks and then gradually decreases to 150 bpm by 14 weeks[115–118]. The early increase in heart rate coincides with the morphological development of the heart, and the subsequent decrease may be the result of functional maturation of the parasympathetic system[116,118,119].

The tachycardia in Turner syndrome and trisomy 13 fetuses may be due to a delay in the functional maturation of the parasympathetic system, resulting in a delay in the physiological decrease in heart rate with gestation after 9 weeks. Alternatively, the higher heart rate of such fetuses represents a compensatory response to the heart strain that may also be responsible for the increased nuchal translucency[120]. In fetal life, the heart normally performs near the peak of the Frank–Starling curve of ventricular function[121] and therefore compensatory increase in cardiac output can only be achieved by relative tachycardia[122]. Maximum tachycardia may be reached, with early heart failure offering an explanation for the lack of a significant association between the extent of increase in nuchal translucency thickness and fetal heart rate. The same hypothesis may also be advanced for the observed mild increase in heart rate of trisomy 21 fetuses.

The relative bradycardia of trisomy 18 fetuses may be related to the fact that, in this chromosomal abnormality, there is early onset growth restriction and the developmental delay is more severe than in trisomies 21 and 13; in such fetuses, the maturation in heart rate would be equivalent to about 8 weeks of gestation. Triploidy is associated with a high rate of early intrauterine lethality and the observed bradycardia in some of these fetuses may represent a preterminal event.

DOPPLER ULTRASOUND FINDINGS IN CHROMOSOMALLY ABNORMAL FETUSES

Umbilical artery

Doppler ultrasound studies have demonstrated that impedance to flow (measured as pulsatility index) decreases with gestation[123,124]. This decrease is believed to be a consequence of the increase in the number of vessels (and their relative volume) within the chorionic villi and the expansion of the intervillous circulation[125].

There is contradictory evidence on the possible association of trisomy 21 at 11–14 weeks of gestation and increased umbilical artery pulsatility index. Martinez et al. reported that the umbilical artery pulsatility index was above the 95th centile in 55% of their nine cases of trisomy 21 and this was not always associated with an increased nuchal translucency; they estimated that the measurements of both factors might allow detection of up to 89% of cases of trisomy 21[126]. In contrast, Jauniaux et al. examined 11 cases of trisomy 21 and reported that there was no significant difference in umbilical artery pulsatility index compared to normal fetuses and that in none of their cases was the pulsatility index above the 95th centile[127]. Similarly, Brown et al. examined 19 trisomy 21 fetuses with increased nuchal translucency at 11–14 weeks and reported that the umbilical artery pulsatility index was not significantly different from normal; the pulsatility index was above the 95th centile in only two of the cases[124].

Umbilical vein

In normal second- and third-trimester fetuses, pulsatile umbilical venous flow is observed only during fetal breathing. Pulsatile venous flow is also observed in fetuses with growth restriction and in non-immune hydrops and is considered to be a late and ominous sign of fetal compromise[128,129]. Evidence from growth-restricted human fetuses and animal models suggests that pulsatile venous flow may result from an increased reversal of flow in the inferior vena cava during atrial contraction, associated with heart failure and abnormal cardiac filling[129,130].

A Doppler study at 11–14 weeks of gestation reported the presence of pulsatile flow in the umbilical vein in about 25% of 302 chromosomally normal fetuses and in 90% of 18 fetuses with trisomy 18 or 13; in 18 fetuses with trisomy 21, the prevalence of pulsatile venous flow was not significantly different from that in chromosomally normal fetuses, but in trisomies 13 and 18 the prevalence was increased[131].

Ductus venosus

The ductus venosus is a unique shunt that carries well-oxygenated blood from the umbilical vein through the inferior atrial inlet on its way across the foramen ovale. It appears to be the most useful vessel in assessing disturbed cardiac function[132]. Blood flow in the ductus is characterized by high velocity during ventricular systole (S-wave) and diastole (D-wave) and by the presence of forward flow during atrial contraction (A-wave). In cardiac failure, with or without cardiac defects, there is absent or reversed A-wave (see Chapter 3, page 102)[133].

It is possible to assess ductus venosus blood flow at 11–14 weeks of gestation by Doppler ultrasound, both transabdominally and transvaginally. A right ventral mid-sagittal plane of the fetal trunk is first obtained during fetal quiescence and the pulsed Doppler gate is placed in the distal portion of the umbilical sinus. The inferior vena cava, left and medial hepatic veins and the ductus venosus drain into a common sub-diaphragmatic vestibulum and therefore, when attempting to obtain flow velocity waveforms from the ductus, care should be taken to avoid contamination from the other veins.

A study, examining ductal flow at 11–14 weeks in fetuses with increased nuchal translucency, reported absent or reversed flow during atrial contraction in 57 of 63 (90.5%) chromosomally abnormal fetuses and in only 13 of 423 (3.1%) chromosomally normal fetuses[134]. In seven of the 13 chromosomally normal fetuses with absent or reversed flow, an ultrasound scan at 14–16 weeks demonstrated a major cardiac defect[134].

Examination of ductal flow is time-consuming and requires skilled operators. It is therefore unlikely that this assessment will be incorporated into the routine first-trimester scan. However, the data suggest that the assessment of ductal flow can potentially play a major role as a secondary method of screening in order to achieve a major reduction in the false-positive rate of primary screening for chromosomal abnormalities by a combination of maternal age, fetal nuchal translucency and maternal serum free β-hCG and PAPP-A at 11–14 weeks. A policy of reserving invasive testing only for those with abnormal ductal flow could reduce the overall need for chorionic villus sampling from 5% to less than 0.5%, with a small reduction (5–10%) in the estimated sensitivity of 90%[134].

NUCHAL TRANSLUCENCY AND MATERNAL SERUM BIOCHEMISTRY

In trisomy 21 during the first trimester of pregnancy, the maternal serum concentration of free β-hCG is higher than in chromosomally normal fetuses (Table 12), whereas PAPP-A is lower (Table 13). Pregnancy-specific β-1 glycoprotein (SP1), α-fetoprotein and inhibin-A do not provide a useful distinction between affected and normal pregnancies[135–137].

Table 12   Median MoM in published studies of free β-hCG in trisomy 21 pregnancies

Study	n	Median MoM	Gestation (weeks)
Ozturk et al. 1990[138]	9	1.62	9–12
Spencer et al. 1992[139]	13	1.85	7–13
Isles et al. 1993[140]	25	1.52	8–14
Macri et al. 1993[141]	25	2.34	9–13
Pescia et al. 1993[142]	5	2.03	8–12
Brambati et al. 1994[143]	13	1.13	8–12
Kellner et al. 1994[144]	5	2.20	8–14
Forest et al. 1997[145]	18	1.92	9–13
Macintosh et al. 1994[146]	21	2.10	8–14
Biagiotti et al. 1995[147]	41	2.00	8–12
Brizot et al. 1995[148]	41	2.00	10–13
Noble et al. 1995[149]	61	2.13	10–13
Krantz et al. 1996[150]	22	2.09	10–13
Scott et al. 1996[151]	8	2.00	10–13
Wald et al. 1996[152]	77	1.79	8–14
Berry et al. 1997[153]	54	1.99	7–13
Spencer et al. 1997[154]	22	1.72	10–13
Haddow et al. 1998[155]	48	2.08	9–13
Wheeler et al. 1998[156]	17	2.06	9–12
de Graaf et al. 1999[157]	37	1.88	—
Spencer et al. 1999[158]	210	2.15	10–14
All studies	772	2.00	

Maternal serum free β-hCG

Maternal serum free β-hCG normally decreases with gestation after 10 weeks. In trisomy 21 pregnancies, the levels are increased and the difference between these and those of normal pregnancies increases with advancing gestation. This may account for the variation in the reported median MoM between the various studies (Table 12)[138–158], because there was a considerable variation in the gestational age range of the populations that were examined. Consequently, population parameters derived from studies using a wide gestational age range are not appropriate if screening is to be focused on the optimal time for nuchal translucency measurement (11–14 weeks). The increase with gestation in the difference between trisomy 21 and normal pregnancies has also been shown in studies of paired samples from trisomy 21 pregnancies collected in the first and second trimesters[153]. In a study involving 210 trisomy 21 pregnancies that were examined at 10–14 weeks, the median free β-hCG was 2.15 MoM (95% CI, 1.94–2.33); at a 5% screen-positive rate, the detection rate using free β-hCG alone is about 35% and, in combination with maternal age, the detection increases to about 45%[158].

Maternal serum PAPP-A

Maternal serum PAPP-A normally increases with gestation. In trisomy 21 pregnancies, the levels are lower but the difference between trisomy 21 and normal pregnancies decreases with advancing gestation. This may account for the variation in the reported median MoM between the various studies (Table 13)[140,143,145,146,150,152,153,155–166]. In a study involving 210 trisomy 21 pregnancies that were examined at 10–14 weeks, the median PAPP-A was 0.51 MoM (95% CI, 0.44–0.56); at a 5% screen-positive rate, the detection rate using PAPP-A alone is about 40% and, in combination with maternal age, the detection increases to about 50%[158].

Maternal serum free β-hCG and PAPP-A

When considering to combine biochemical markers, it is necessary to take into account the degree of correlation between the markers. In our study, involving 210 trisomy 21 and 946 chromosomally normal controls, the correlations were 0.216 and 0.160, respectively[158]. Additionally, each marker showed a small but significant negative correlation with maternal weight (PAPP-A, $r = -0.278$; free β-hCG, $r = -0.146$). After combining free β-hCG and PAPP-A with maternal age in mathematical models, it has been estimated that the detection rate of trisomy 21 is about 60% at a 5% screen-positive rate (Table 14)[150,152,153,155–158,167,168].

Table 13 Median MoM in published studies of PAPP-A in trisomy 21 pregnancies

Study	n	Median MoM	Gestation (weeks)
Wald et al. 1992[159]	19	0.23	9–12
Brambati et al. 1993[160]	14	0.27	6–11
Hurley et al. 1993[161]	7	0.33	8–12
Isles et al. 1993[140]	25	0.38	8–14
Muller et al. 1993[162]	17	0.42	10–14
Bersinger et al. 1994[163]	29	0.60	10–13
Brambati et al. 1994[143]	13	0.31	8–12
Brizot et al. 1994[164]	45	0.50	10–13
Macintosh et al. 1994[146]	14	0.34	8–14
Spencer et al. 1994[165]	21	0.62	7–14
Casals et al. 1996[166]	19	0.42	10–13
Krantz et al. 1996[150]	22	0.41	10–13
Wald et al. 1996[152]	77	0.43	8–14
Berry et al. 1997[153]	52	0.50	7–13
Forest et al. 1997[145]	18	0.46	9–13
Haddow et al. 1998[155]	48	0.41	9–13
Wheeler & Sinosich 1998[156]	17	0.43	9–12
de Graaf et al. 1999[157]	37	0.63	—
Spencer et al. 1999[158]	210	0.51	10–14
All studies	704	0.469	

Table 14 Estimated detection rate for trisomy 21 by a combination of maternal age and first-trimester maternal serum PAPP-A and free β-hCG at a 5% fixed screen-positive rate

Study	Trisomy 21	Gestation (weeks)	Detection (%)
Krantz et al. 1996[150]	22	10–13	63
Wald et al. 1996[152]	77	8–14	62
Berry et al. 1997[153]	47	9–14	55
Orlandi et al. 1997[167]	11	9–14	61
Haddow et al. 1998[155]	48	9–15	60
Wheeler & Sinosich 1998[156]	17	9–12	67
de Graaf et al. 1999[157]	37	10–14	55
Spencer et al. 1999[158]	210	10–14	67
Tsukerman et al. 1999[168]	31	8–13	69

Fetal nuchal translucency and maternal serum free β-hCG and PAPP-A

There is no significant association between fetal nuchal translucency and maternal serum free β-hCG or PAPP-A in either trisomy 21 or chromosomally normal pregnancies[147,158,164]. The estimated detection rate for trisomy 21 by a combination of maternal age, fetal nuchal translucency and maternal serum PAPP-A and free β-hCG is about 90% for a screen-positive rate of 5% (Table 15)[148,157,158,164,167,169]. Alternatively, at a fixed detection rate of 70%, the screen-positive rate would be only 1%[158]. The performance of the combined test now requires assessment in prospective studies.

Table 15   Estimated detection rate for trisomy 21 by a combination of maternal age, fetal nuchal translucency and first-trimester maternal serum PAPP-A and free β-hCG at a 5% fixed false-positive rate

Study	Trisomy 21	Gestation (weeks)	Screen-positive (%)	Detection (%)
Brizot *et al.* 1994,1995[148,164]	80	10–14	5.0	89
Orlandi *et al.* 1997[167]	11	9–14	5.0	87
de Graaf *et al.* 1999[157]	37	10–14	5.0	85
De Biasio *et al.* 1999[169]	13	10–14	3.3	85
Spencer *et al.* 1999[158]	210	10–14	5.0	89

One-stop clinics for early assessment of fetal risk

An important development in biochemical analysis is the introduction of a new technique (random access immunoassay analyzer using time-resolved-amplified-cryptate-emission), which provides automated, precise and reproducible measurements within 30 minutes of obtaining a blood sample[158]. This has made it possible to combine biochemical and ultrasonographic testing as well as to counsel in one-stop clinics for early assessment of fetal risk (OSCAR).

NUCHAL TRANSLUCENCY FOLLOWED BY SECOND-TRIMESTER BIOCHEMISTRY

At 16 weeks of gestation, the median maternal serum concentrations of α-fetoprotein, estriol, hCG (total and free β) and inhibin A in trisomy 21 pregnancies are different from normal. The risk for trisomy 21 can be derived by multiplying the *background* maternal age and gestational age-related risk by the likelihood ratios for these substances, after corrections for the interrelations between them. The risk of trisomy 21 is increased if the levels of hCG and/or inhibin A are high, and the levels of α-fetoprotein and/or estriol are low. The estimated detection rates are 50–70% for a screen-positive rate of about 5%.

In women having second-trimester biochemical testing following first-trimester nuchal translucency screening (with or without maternal serum biochemistry), the *background* risk needs to be adjusted to take into account the first-trimester screening results. Since first-trimester screening identifies almost 90% of trisomy 21 pregnancies, second-trimester biochemistry will identify – at best – 6% (60% of the residual 10%) of the affected pregnancies, with doubling of the overall invasive testing rate (from 5% to 10%). It is theoretically possible to use various statistical techniques to combine nuchal translucency with different components of first-trimester and second-trimester biochemical testing. One such hypothetical model has combined first-trimester nuchal and PAPP-A with second-trimester free β-hCG, estriol and inhibin A, claiming a potential sensitivity of 94% for a 5% false-positive rate[170]. Even if the assumptions made in this statistical technique are valid, it is unlikely that it will gain widespread clinical acceptability[171].

Two studies have reported on the impact of first-trimester screening by nuchal translucency on second-trimester serum biochemical testing. In one study, the proportion of affected pregnancies in the screen-positive group (positive predictive value) of screening by the double test in the second trimester was 1 in 40; after the introduction of screening by nuchal translucency, 83% of trisomy 21 pregnancies were identified in the first trimester and the positive predictive value of biochemical screening decreased to 1 in 200[172]. In the second study, first-trimester screening by nuchal translucency identified 71% of trisomy 21 pregnancies for a screen-positive rate of 2%, and the positive predictive value of second-trimester screening by the quadruple test was only 1 in 150[173].

In women who had first-trimester screening by a combination of fetal nuchal translucency and maternal serum PAPP-A and free β-hCG, it is clearly advisable that second-trimester biochemical testing is avoided because, first, the sensitivities of first- and second-trimester biochemical screening are similar; second, the main component of the second-trimester biochemical screening is free β-hCG, and, third, there is a good correlation between first- and second-trimester maternal serum hCG levels. If both first- and second-trimester biochemical testing have been carried out, then the likelihood ratio from the measurement of nuchal translucency can be multiplied with the results of either first- or second-trimester serum testing. This is certainly valid for second-trimester programs that are mainly based on free β-hCG because the interrelation between nuchal translucency and this metabolite has been established[148].

NUCHAL TRANSLUCENCY FOLLOWED BY SECOND-TRIMESTER ULTRASONOGRAPHY

Major chromosomal abnormalities are often associated with multiple fetal defects that can be detected by ultrasound examination. For example, trisomy 21 is associated with a tendency for brachycephaly, mild ventriculomegaly, flattening of the face, nuchal edema, atrioventricular septal defects, duodenal atresia and echogenic bowel, mild hydronephrosis, shortening of the limbs, sandal gap and clinodactyly or mid-phalanx hypoplasia of the fifth finger. Trisomy 18 is associated with strawberry-shaped head, choroid plexus cysts, absent corpus callosum, enlarged cisterna magna, facial cleft, micrognathia, nuchal edema, heart defects, diaphragmatic hernia, esophageal atresia, exomphalos, renal defects, myelomeningocele, growth restriction and shortening of the limbs, radial aplasia, overlapping fingers and talipes or rocker bottom feet.

The overall risk for chromosomal abnormalities increases with the total number of defects that are identified (Figure 17)[174]. It is therefore recommended that, when a defect/marker is detected at routine ultrasound examination, a thorough check is made for the other features of the chromosomal abnormality known to be associated with that marker; should additional defects be identified, the risk is dramatically increased. In the case of apparently isolated defects, the decision of whether to carry out an invasive test depends on the type of defect.

Major defects

If the mid-trimester scan demonstrates major defects, it is advisable to offer fetal karyo-typing, even if these defects are apparently isolated. The prevalence of these defects is

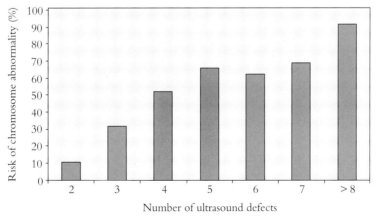

Figure 17   Incidence of chromosomal abnormalities in relation to number of sonographically detected defects[174]

low and therefore the cost implications are small. If the defects are either lethal or they are associated with severe handicap, fetal karyotyping constitutes one of a series of investigations to determine the possible cause and thus the risk of recurrence. Examples of these defects include hydrocephalus, holoprosencephaly, multicystic renal dysplasia and severe hydrops. In the case of isolated neural tube defects, there is controversy as to whether the risk for chromosomal defects is increased. Similarly, for skeletal dysplasias where the likely diagnosis is obvious by ultrasonography, it would probably be unnecessary to perform karyotyping. If the defect is potentially correctable by intrauterine or postnatal surgery, it may be logical to exclude an underlying chromosomal abnormality – especially because, for many of these conditions, the usual abnormality is trisomy 18 or 13. Examples include facial cleft, diaphragmatic hernia, esophageal atresia, exomphalos and many of the cardiac defects. In the case of isolated gastroschisis or small bowel obstruction, there is no evidence of increased risk of trisomies.

Minor defects or markers

These defects are common and they are not usually associated with any handicap, unless there is an associated chromosomal abnormality. Routine karyotyping of all pregnancies with these markers would have major implications, both in terms of miscarriage and in economic costs. It is best to base counselling on an individual estimated risk for a chromosomal abnormality, rather than the arbitrary advice that invasive testing is recommended because the risk is 'high'. The estimated risk can be derived by multiplying the *background risk* (based on maternal age, gestational age, history of previously affected pregnancies and, where appropriate, the results of previous screening by nuchal translucency and/or biochemistry in the current pregnancy) by the likelihood ratio of the specific defect[175–177]. For the following conditions, there are sufficient data in the literature to estimate the likelihood ratio for trisomy 21.

Nuchal edema or fold of more than 6 mm

This is the second-trimester form of nuchal translucency. It is found in about 0.5% of fetuses and it may be of no pathological significance. However, it is sometimes associated with chromosomal defects, cardiac anomalies, infection or genetic syndromes[46]. For isolated nuchal edema, the risk for trisomy 21 may be 15 times the background[178,179].

Short femur

If the femur is below the 5th centile and all other measurements are normal, the baby is likely to be normal but rather short. Rarely is this a sign of dwarfism. Occasionally, it may be a marker of chromosomal defects. On the basis of existing studies, short femur is found four times as commonly in trisomy 21 fetuses compared to normal fetuses[180–185]. However, there is some evidence that isolated short femur may not be more common in trisomic than in normal fetuses[178].

Hyperechogenic bowel

This is found in about 0.5% of fetuses and is usually of no pathological significance. The commonest cause is intra-amniotic bleeding, but occasionally it may be a marker of cystic fibrosis or chromosomal defects. For isolated hyperechogenic bowel, the risk for trisomy 21 may be three times the background[178,186,187].

Echogenic foci in the heart

These are found in about 4% of pregnancies and they are usually of no pathological significance. However, they are sometimes associated with cardiac defects and chromosomal abnormalities. For isolated hyperechogenic foci the risk, for trisomy 21 may be four-times the background[178,189–191].

Choroid plexus cysts

These are found in about 1–2% of pregnancies and they are usually of no pathological significance. When other defects are present, there is a high risk of chromosomal defects, usually trisomy 18 but occasionally trisomy 21. For isolated choroid plexus cysts, the risk for trisomy 18 and trisomy 21 is about 1.5 times the background[177].

Mild hydronephrosis

This is found in about 1–2% of pregnancies and is usually of no pathological significance. When other abnormalities are present, there is a high risk of chromosomal defects, usually trisomy 21. For isolated mild hydronephrosis, the risk for trisomy 21 is about 1.5 times the background[176,192,193].

There are no data on the interrelation between these second-trimester ultrasound markers and nuchal translucency at 11–14 weeks or first- and second-trimester biochemistry. However, there is no obvious physiological reason for such an interrelation and it is therefore reasonable to assume that they are independent. Consequently, in estimating the risk in a pregnancy with a marker, it is logical to take into account the results of previous screening tests. For example, in a 20-year-old woman at 20 weeks of gestation (background risk of 1 in 1295), who had a 11–14 week assessment by nuchal translucency measurement that resulted in a 5-fold reduction in risk (to about 1 in 6475), after the diagnosis of mild hydronephrosis at the 20-week scan, the estimated risk has increased by a factor of 1.5 to 1 in 4317. In contrast, for the same ultrasound finding of fetal mild hydronephrosis in a 40-year-old woman (background risk of 1 in 82), who did not have nuchal translucency or biochemistry screening, the new estimated risk is 1 in 55.

There are some exceptions to this process of *sequential screening,* which assumes independence between the findings of different screening results. The findings of nuchal edema or a cardiac defect at the mid-trimester scan cannot be considered independently of nuchal translucency screening at 11–14 weeks. Similarly, hyperechogenic bowel (which may be due to intra-amniotic bleeding) and relative shortening of the femur (which may be due to placental insufficiency) may well be related to serum biochemistry (high free β-hCG and inhibin-A and low estriol may be markers of placental damage) and can therefore not be considered independently in estimating the risk for trisomy 21. For example, in a 20-year-old woman (background risk for trisomy 21 of 1 in 1295), with high free β-hCG and inhibin-A and low estriol at the 16-week serum testing resulting in a 10-fold increase in risk (to 1 in 129), the finding of hyperechogenic bowel at the 20-week scan should not lead to the erroneous conclusion of a further three-fold increase in risk (to 1 in 43). The coincidence of biochemical and sonographic features of placental insufficiency makes it very unlikely that the problem is trisomy 21 and should lead to increased monitoring for pre-eclampsia and growth restriction, rather than amniocentesis for fetal karyotyping.

NON-INVASIVE DIAGNOSIS USING FETAL CELLS FROM MATERNAL BLOOD

During the last 30 years, extensive research has aimed at developing a non-invasive method for prenatal diagnosis based on the isolation and examination of fetal cells found in the maternal circulation. Erythroblasts have attracted most attention because they are abundant in early fetal blood; they are extremely rare in normal adult blood and their half-life in adult blood is only about 30 days. Trophoblastic cells entering the maternal circulation are cleared by the maternal lungs and are therefore not useful candidates for prenatal diagnosis. Fetal white blood cells are present in maternal blood but their number is very low and they have a very long half-life (about 5 years), which may therefore lead to contamination from previous pregnancies.

About 1 in 10^3–10^7 nucleated cells in maternal blood are fetal[194–196]. The proportion of fetal cells can be enriched to about 1 in 10–100 by techniques such as magnetic cell sorting (MACS) or fluorescence activated cell sorting (FACS) after attachment of magnetically labelled or fluorescent antibodies on to specific fetal cell surface markers[194,197–199]. The most commonly used antibody is anti-CD71, which is directed against the transferrin receptor present on the surface of all cells actively incorporating iron[198,200]. Other cell types in maternal blood, such as activated lymphocytes, have this receptor but anti-CD71 provides a reasonable level of enrichment once maternal lymphocytes have been removed. Magnetic cell sorting is cheaper, quicker and requires less expertise to perform than FACS. The technique utilizes metallic beads labelled with an antibody specific for the target cell. The antibody is incubated with the sample and the cell–antibody–bead complex is isolated by placing on a magnet. Successful use of MACS involves prior separation of cells by triple density centrifugation. Essentially, the maternal blood sample is placed in a tube containing three sugar-based reagents of different density and, after centrifugation, the middle layer containing erythroblasts and neutrophil granulocytes is separated. These cells are incubated with magnetically labelled CD71 antibody and MACS is then carried out (Figure 18).

The resulting sample is unsuitable for traditional cytogenetic analysis because it is still highly contaminated with maternal cells. However, with the use of chromo-some-specific DNA probes and fluorescent *in situ* hybridization (FISH), it is possible to suspect fetal trisomy by the presence of three-signal nuclei in some of the cells of the maternal blood enriched for fetal cells. It is now possible to identify simultaneously all major chromosomal abnormalities by the use of multicolor probes directed against chromosomes 21, 18, 13, Y and X in interphase nuclei (Figure 19). One of the major problems with FISH is that 1–2% of normal diploid cells give three-signal nuclei and about 10–20% of trisomic cells give two-signal nuclei[201].

Bianchi *et al.* detected three-signal nuclei from a trisomy 21 pregnancy after enrichment for fetal cells in maternal blood by FACS[202]. Ganshirt-Ahlert *et al.* found three-signal nuclei in 9–17% of cells from ten trisomy 21 and six trisomy 18 pregnancies after sorting by MACS; in ten chromosomally normal pregnancies, 0–7% of cells had three-signal nuclei[203]. Simpson and Elias reported the presence of three-signal nuclei, after sorting by FACS, in 2.8–74% of cells from five trisomy 21 and two trisomy 18 pregnancies, but in none of 61 chromosomally normal pregnancies[204].

Al-Mufti *et al.* took maternal peripheral blood immediately before chorionic villus sampling from 230 women with singleton pregnancies at 11–14 weeks of gestation[199]. These pregnancies had been identified as being at high risk for trisomies after screening by a combination of maternal age and fetal nuchal translucency thickness. Triple density gradient centrifugation, followed by incubation of the erythroblast-rich fraction with magnetically labelled CD71 antibody, MACS and FISH were carried out. In 3% of cases, no fetal hemoglobin-positive cells were observed. In the chromosomally abnormal group, the percentage of cells demonstrating three-signal nuclei was higher than in the normal group but there was an overlap in values between the two groups (Figure 20).

Using a 21-chromosome-specific probe, three-signal nuclei were present in at least 5% of the enriched cells from 61% of the trisomy 21 pregnancies and in none of the normal pregnancies. For a cut-off of 3% of three-signal nuclei, the sensitivity for

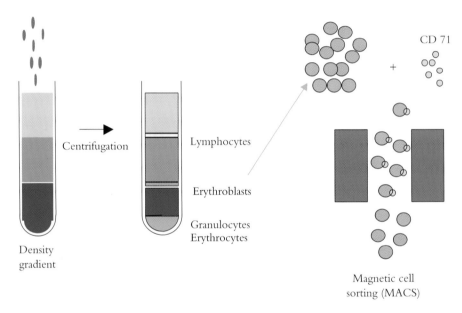

Figure 18 Triple density centrifugation and magnetic cell sorting techniques, using magnetically labelled anti-CD71 (antibody against transferrin receptor antigen)

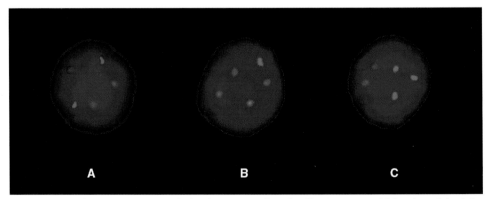

Figure 19 Fluorescence *in situ* hybridization analyzed cells, in maternal blood enriched for fetal cells, from trisomy 21 (A), trisomy 18 (B) and trisomy 13 (C). Pregnancies demonstrating three-signal nuclei with the appropriate chromosome-specific probe

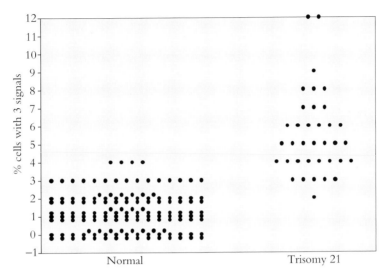

Figure 20 Percentage of cells with three-signal nuclei using the 21 chromosome-specific probe in maternal blood enriched for fetal cells from chromosomally normal pregnancies and those with trisomy 21

trisomy 21 was 97% for a false-positive rate of 13%. Similar values were obtained in trisomies 18 and 13 using the appropriate chromosome-specific probe (Table 16).

The findings that, with the 21-chromosome-specific probe, three-signal nuclei were present in at least 5% of the enriched cells from about 60% of trisomy 21 pregnancies and in none of the normal pregnancies, suggest that this method could be associated with the same rate of detection of trisomy 21 as second-trimester serum biochemistry but with the advantage that the invasive testing rate may be as low as 0% rather than 5%. However, unlike serum biochemistry testing, which is relatively

Table 16 Sensitivity and false-positive rate for the various cut-off percentages of cells with three-signal nuclei in the chromosomally abnormal and normal groups using fluorescent probes for chromosomes 21, 18 and 13

	Chromosome 21 probe		Chromosome 18 probe		Chromosome 13 probe	
Cut-off	Trisomy 21 (n = 36)	Normal (n = 142)	Trisomy 18 (n = 24)	Normal (n = 1342)	Trisomy 13 (n = 10)	Normal (n = 142)
≥ 3%	35 (97.22%)	19 (13.38%)	23 (95.83%)	23 (16.2%)	10 (100%)	32 (22.5%)
≥ 4%	30 (83.33%)	4 (2.8%)	20 (83.30%)	9 (6.34%)	8 (80%)	7 (4.93%)
≥ 5%	22 (61.11%)	0	13 (54.16%)	0	5 (50%)	0

easy to apply for mass population screening, enrichment of fetal cells by triple density gradient centrifugation and MACS, followed by FISH, is both labor intensive and requires highly skilled operators. In the case of FISH, there are promising developments for automated computerized analysis of cells which are likely to simplify processing of the slides. The extent to which the techniques for enrichment of fetal cells could be improved, to achieve a higher yield of the necessary cells, as well as become automated, to allow simultaneous analysis of a large number of samples, remains to be seen.

On the basis of currently available technology, examination of fetal cells from maternal peripheral blood is more likely to find an application as a method for assessment of risk, rather than the non–invasive prenatal diagnosis of chromosomal defects. First-line screening by a combination of maternal age, fetal nuchal translucency and maternal serum free β-hCG with PAPP-A could detect 90% of trisomy 21 pregnancies for an invasive testing rate of about 5%[158]. One option in the management of the high-risk group is to carry out FISH on maternal blood enriched for fetal cells and reserve chorionic villus sampling only for those pregnancies where no fetal hemoglobin-positive cells are recovered and those where at least 3% of the cells demonstrate three signals with the 21-chromosome specific probe. Such a policy could potentially reduce the need for invasive testing to less than 1% of the whole population with a minor loss (about 3%) in the sensitivity for detection of trisomy 21.

INVASIVE DIAGNOSIS OF CHROMOSOMAL DEFECTS

Amniocentesis

The feasibility of culturing and karyotyping amniotic fluid cells was first demonstrated in the late 1960s[32,33]. Early attempts at genetic amniocentesis were made transvaginally, but subsequently the transabdominal approach was adopted. In the early 1970s, amniocentesis was performed 'blindly'. In the late 1970s and early 1980s, ultrasound, initially static and subsequently real-time, was used to identify a placenta-free area for entry into a pocket of amniotic fluid. The position of this was marked on the maternal abdomen and, after a variable length of time, in some studies up to 2 days, the operator would 'blindly' insert the needle. It is therefore not surprising that early reports on the use of ultrasound produced conflicting conclusions, with some suggesting that it was actually detrimental. Amniocentesis is now performed with continuous ultrasound guidance.

Ager and Oliver reported a critical appraisal of all the studies on amniocentesis that were published during 1975–85[205]. There were 28 major national studies, each involving at least 1000 cases; the total post-amniocentesis fetal loss rate, including spontaneous abortion, intrauterine death and neonatal death was 2.4–5.2%. In four of the 28 studies, there were matched controls that did not undergo amniocentesis; the total fetal loss rate was 1.8–3.7%. On the basis of these data it was estimated that the procedure-related risk of fetal loss from amniocentesis was 0.2–2.1%[205].

The only randomized trial was performed in Denmark[206]. In this study, 4606 low-risk, healthy women, 25–34 years old, at 14–20 weeks of gestation, were randomly allocated to amniocentesis or ultrasound examination alone. The total fetal loss rate in the patients having amniocentesis was 1% higher than in the controls. There were significant associations between spontaneous fetal loss and (1) puncture of the placenta, (2) high maternal serum α-fetoprotein and (3) discolored amniotic fluid. The Danish study also reported that amniocentesis was associated with an increased risk of respiratory distress syndrome and pneumonia in neonates. Some studies have reported an increased incidence of talipes and dislocation of the hip after amniocentesis, but this was not confirmed by the Danish study[206].

Early amniocentesis

In the late 1980s, early amniocentesis was introduced and studies with complete pregnancy follow-up have reported that the procedure-related fetal loss rate was around 3–6%.

A prospective study involving 1301 singleton pregnancies compared early amniocentesis with chorionic villus sampling at 10–13 weeks of gestation[207]. The procedures were performed (1) for the same indication, (2) at the same gestational range, (3) by the same group of operators, (4) using essentially the same technique of transabdominal ultrasound-guided insertion of a 20-G needle, and (5) the samples were sent to the same laboratories. Successful samplings resulting in a non-mosaic cytogenetic result were the same for both early amniocentesis and chorionic villus sampling (97.5%). Furthermore, the intervals between sampling and obtaining results were similar for the two techniques. The main indication for repeat testing in the chorionic villus sampling group was mosaicism, whereas, in the early amniocentesis group, it was failed culture; this failure was related to gestation at sampling: 5.3% at 10 weeks and 1.6% at 11–13 weeks. Spontaneous loss (intrauterine and neonatal death) after early amniocentesis was approximately 3% higher than after chorionic villus sampling. The gestation at delivery and birth weight of the infants were similar after both procedures, and the frequencies of preterm delivery or low birth weight were not higher than those that would be expected in a normal population. In the early amniocentesis group, the incidence of talipes equinovarus (1.63%) was higher than in the chorionic villus sampling group (0.56%)[207].

A randomized study in Denmark involving 1160 pregnancies compared trans-abdominal chorionic villus sampling at 10–12 weeks with early amniocentesis at 11–13 weeks using a filtration technique; randomization was at 10 weeks[208]. Fetal loss after chorionic villus sampling was 4.8% and after early amniocentesis it was 5.4%, but this difference was not significant. The study was stopped early because interim analysis of results demonstrated a significantly higher rate of talipes equinovarus (1.7%) after early amniocentesis than after chorionic villus sampling (0%)[208].

A randomized study in Canada involving 4374 pregnancies compared early amniocentesis at 11–13 weeks with amniocentesis at 15–17 weeks using a 22-G needle; randomization was at 9–12 weeks[209]. Total fetal loss in the early amniocentesis group (7.6%) was significantly higher than in the late amniocentesis group (5.9%). Furthermore, early amniocentesis was associated with a significantly higher incidence of talipes (1.3% compared to 0.1%) and postprocedural amniotic fluid leakage (3.5% compared to 1.7%)[209].

On the basis of existing data, it is therefore clear that amniocentesis should not be carried out before 13 weeks of gestation. The extent to which early amniocentesis performed after 13 weeks will prove to be safer than chorionic villus sampling is currently under investigation by an NIH-sponsored study in the USA.

Chorionic villus sampling

Chorionic villus sampling was first attempted in the late 1960s by hysteroscopy, but the technique was associated with low success in both sampling and karyotyping and was abandoned in favor of amniocentesis. In the 1970s, the desire for early diagnosis led to the revival of chorionic villus sampling, which was initially carried out by aspiration via a cannula that was introduced 'blindly' into the uterus through the cervix. Subsequently, ultrasound guidance was used for the transcervical or transabdominal insertion of a variety of cannulas or biopsy forceps.

Four randomized studies have examined the rate of fetal loss following first-trimester chorionic villus sampling compared to that of amniocentesis at 16 weeks of gestation (Table 17)[210–213]. In total, about 10 000 pregnancies were examined and the results demonstrated that, in centers experienced in both procedures, fetal loss is no greater after first-trimester chorionic villus sampling compared to second-trimester amniocentesis. The most likely explanation for the increased loss after chorionic villus sampling in the European study is the participation of many centers with little experience in this technique.

Table 17 Total fetal loss rate in four randomized studies comparing first-trimester chorionic villus sampling with second-trimester amniocentesis

Study	n	Chorionic villus sampling	Amniocentesis
Canadian study[210]	2787	7.6%	7.1%
Danish study[211]	3079	6.3%	7.0%
Finnish study[212]	800	6.3%	6.4%
European study[213]	3248	14.0%*	9.0%

*$p < 0.01$

In 1991, severe transverse limb abnormalities, micrognathia and microglossia were reported in five of 289 pregnancies that had undergone chorionic villus sampling at less than 10 weeks of gestation[214]. Subsequently, a series of other reports confirmed the possible association between early chorionic villus sampling and fetal defects; analysis of 75 such cases demonstrated a strong association between the severity of the defect and the gestation at sampling[215]. Thus, the median gestation at chorionic villus sampling was 8 weeks for those with amputation of the whole limb and 10 weeks for those with defects affecting the terminal phalanxes. The background incidence of terminal transverse limb defects is about 1.8 per 10 000 live births[216], and the incidence following early chorionic villus sampling is estimated at 1 in 200–1000 cases. The types of defects are compatible with the pattern of limb development, which is essentially completed by the 10th week of gestation. Possible mechanisms by which early sampling may lead to limb defects include hypoperfusion, embolization or release of vasoactive substances, and all these mechanisms are related to trauma. It is therefore imperative that chorionic villus sampling is performed only after 11 weeks by appropriately trained operators. The data from the International Registry on chorionic villus sampling are disputing the association between this procedure and limb reduction defects[217].

REFERENCES

1. Langdon Down J. Observations on an ethnic classification of idiots. *Clin Lectures and Reports*, London Hospital 1866; 3:259–62
2. Crookshank FG. In *The Mongol in our Midst*. London: Kegan Paul, Trench and Trubner Ltd, 1924
3. Fraser J, Mitchell A. Kalmuc idiocy: report of a case with autopsy with notes on 62 cases by A. Mitchell. *J Ment Sci* 1876;22:169–79
4. Goddard HH. In *Feeble-mindedness, its Causes and Consequences*. New York: Macmillan and Co, 1914
5. Sutherland GA. Mongolian imbecility in infants. *Practitioner* 1899;63:632
6. Shuttleworth GE. Mongolian imbecility. *Br Med J* 1909;2:661–5

7. Cafferata JF. Contribution a la literature du mongolisme. *Arch Med Enf* 1909;12:929

8. Caldecott C. Tuberculosis as a cause of death in mongolism. *Br Med J* 1909;2:665

9. Tredgold AF. In *Mental Deficiency (Amentia)*. London: Bailliere, Tindall and Cox, 1908

10. Stoeltzner W. Zur Atiologie des Mongolismus. *Munich Med Wschr* 1919;66:1943

11. Vas J. Beitrage zur Pathogenese und Therapie der Idiotia Mongoliana. *Jb Kinderheik* 1925;111:51

12. Benda CE, Bixby EM. Function of the thyroid and the pituitary in mongolism. *Am J Dis Child* 1939;58:1240

13. Barnes NP. Mongolism – importance of early recognition and treatment. *Ann Clin Med* 1923;1:302

14. Jenkins RL. Etiology of mongolism. *Am J Dis Child* 1933;45:506

15. Rosanoff AJ, Handy LM. Etiology of mongolism with special reference to its occurrence in twins. *Am J Dis Child* 1934;48:764

16. Bleyer A. Indications that mongoloid idiocy is a gametic mutation of degenerative type. *Am J Dis Child* 1934;47:342

17. Halbertsma T. Mongolism in one of twins and the etiology of mongolism. *Am J Dis Child* 1923;25:350

18. Lelong M, Borniche P, Kreisler L, Baudy R. Mongolien issu de mere mongolienne. *Arch Franc Pediat* 1949; 6:231

19. Rehn AT, Thomas E. Family history of a mongolian girl who bore a mongolian child. *Am J Ment Defic* 1957;62:496

20. Penrose LS. Maternal age in familial mongolism. *J Ment Sci* 1951;97:738

21. Penrose LS. Mongolian idiocy (mongolism) and maternal age. *Ann NY Acad Sci* 1953;57:494

22. Waardenburg PJ. In *Das menschliche Auge und seine Erbalagen*. Haag: Martinus Nijhoff, 1932

23. Tijo JH, Levan A. The chromosome number of man. *Hereditas* 1956;42:1

24. Ford CE, Hamerton JL. The chromosomes of man. *Nature* 1956;168:1020

25. Lejeune J, Gautier M, Turpin R. Etudes des chromosomes somatiques de neuf enfants mongoliens. *C R Acad Sci* 1959;248:1721

26. Jacobs PA, Baikie AG, Court Brown WM, Strong JA. The somatic chromosomes in mongolism. *Lancet* 1959;1:710

27. Polani PE, Briggs JH, Ford CE, Clarke CM, Berg JM. A mongol girl with 46 chromosomes. *Lancet* 1960;1:721

28. Penrose LS, Ellis JR, Delhanty JDA. Chromosomal translocations on mongolism and in normal relatives. *Lancet* 1960;2:409

29. Clarke CM, Edwards JH, Smallpiece V. 21 trisomy/normal mosaicism in an intelligent child with mongoloid characters. *Lancet* 1961;1:1028

30. Antonarakis SE, Lewi JG, Adelsberger PA, Petersen MB, Schinzel AA, Cohen MM, Roulston D, Schwartz S, Mikkelsen M, Tranebjorg L, Greenberg F, How DI, Rudd NL. Parental origin of the extra chromosome in trisomy 21 as indicated by analysis of DNA polymorphisms. *N Engl J Med* 1991;324:872–6

31. Korenberg JR. Toward a molecular understanding of Down syndrome. *Prog Clin Bio Res* 1993;384:87–115

32. Steele MW, Breg WR. Chromosome analysis of human amniotic-fluid cells. *Lancet* 1966;i:383–5

33. Valenti C, Schutta EJ, Kehaty T. Prenatal diagnosis of Down's syndrome. *Lancet* 1968;ii:220

34. Snijders RJM, Nicolaides KH. Assessment of risks. In *Ultrasound Markers for Fetal Chromosomal Defects*. Carnforth, UK: Parthenon Publishing, 1996:109–13

35. Koulisher L, Gillerot Y. Down's syndrome in Wallonia (South Belgium), 1971–1978: cytogenetics and incidence. *Hum Genet* 1980;54:243–50

36. Hook EB, Lindsjo A. Down syndrome in live births by single year maternal age interval in a Swedish study: comparison with results from a New York State study. *Am J Hum Genet* 1978;30:19–27

37. Hecht CA, Hook EB. The imprecision in rates of Down syndrome by 1-year maternal age intervals: a critical analysis of rates used in biochemical screening. *Prenat Diagn* 1994;14:729–38

38. Snijders RJM, Sundberg K, Holzgreve W, Henry G, Nicolaides KH. Maternal age and gestation-specific risk for trisomy 21. *Ultrasound Obstet Gynecol* 1999;13:167–70

39. Snijders RJM, Holzgreve W, Cuckle H, Nicolaides KH. Maternal age-specific risks for trisomies at 9–14 weeks' gestation. *Prenat Diagn* 1994;14:543–52

40. Snijders RJM, Sebire NJ, Cuckle H, Nicolaides KH. Maternal age and gestational age-specific risks for chromosomal defects. *Fetal Diag Ther* 1995;10:356–67

41. Halliday JL, Watson LF, Lumley J, Danks DM, Sheffield LJ. New estimates of Down syndrome risks at chorionic villus sampling, amniocentesis, and livebirth in women of advanced maternal age from a uniquely defined population. *Prenat Diagn* 1995; 15:455–65

42. Morris JK, Wald NJ, Watt HC. Fetal loss in Down syndrome pregnancies. *Prenat Diagn* 1999;19:142–5

43. Macintosh MC, Wald NJ, Chard T, Hansen J, Mikkelsen M, Therkelsen AJ, Petersen GB, Lundsteen C. Selective miscarriage of Down's syndrome fetuses in women aged 35 years and older. *Br J Obstet Gynaecol* 1995;102:798–801

44. Snijders RJM, Sundberg K, Holzgreve W, Henry G, Nicolaides KH. Maternal age and gestation-specific risk for trisomy 21: effect of previous affected pregnancy. In press

45. Azar G, Snijders RJM, Gosden CM, Nicolaides KH. Fetal nuchal cystic hygromata: associated malformations and chromosomal defects. *Fetal Diagn Ther* 1991;6:46–57

46. Nicolaides KH, Azar G, Snijders RJM, Gosden CM. Fetal nuchal edema: associated malformations and chromosomal defects. *Fetal Diagn Ther* 1992;7:123–31

47. Whitlow BJ, Economides DL. The optimal gestational age to examine fetal anatomy and measure nuchal translucency in the first trimester. *Ultrasound Obstet Gynecol* 1998;11:258–61

48. Braithwaite JM, Economides DL. The measurement of nuchal translucency with transabdominal and transvaginal sonography – success rates, repeatability and levels of agreement. *Br J Radiol* 1995; 68:720–3

49. Braithwaite JM, Morris RW, Economides DL. Nuchal translucency measurements: frequency distribution and changes with gestation in a general population. *Br J Obstet Gynaecol* 1996;103:1201–4

50. Whitlow BJ, Chatzipapas IK, Economides DL. The effect of fetal neck position on nuchal translucency measurement. *Br J Obstet Gynaecol* 1998;105:872–6

51. Schaefer M, Laurichesse-Delmas H, Ville Y. The effect of nuchal cord on nuchal translucency measurement at 10–14 weeks. *Ultrasound Obstet Gynecol* 1998;11:271–3

52. Herman A, Maymon R, Dreazen E, Caspi E, Bukovsky I, Weinraub Z. Nuchal translucency audit: a novel image-scoring method. *Ultrasound Obstet Gynecol* 1998;12:398–403

53. Braithwaite JM, Kadir RA, Pepera TA, Morris RW, Thompson PJ, Economides DL. Nuchal translucency measurement: training of potential examiners. *Ultrasound Obstet Gynecol* 1996;8:192–5

54. Bower S, Chitty L, Bewley S, Roberts L, Clark T, Fisk NM, Maxwell D, Rodeck CH. First trimester nuchal translucency screening of the general population: data from three centres [abstract].

Presented at the *27th British Congress of Obstetrics and Gynaecology*. Dublin: Royal College of Obstetrics and Gynaecology, 1995

55. Roberts LJ, Bewley S, Mackinson AM, Rodeck CH. First trimester fetal nuchal translucency: Problems with screening the general population 1. *Br J Obstet Gynaecol* 1995;102:381–5

56. Monni G, Zoppi MA, Ibba RM, Floris M. Results of measurement of nuchal translucency before and after training. (Letter in reply to: Assessment of fetal nuchal translucency test for Down's syndrome. *Lancet* 1997, 350:745–55). *Lancet* 1997;350:1631

57. Pandya PP, Altman D, Brizot ML, Pettersen H, Nicolaides KH. Repeatability of measurement of fetal nuchal translucency thickness. *Ultrasound Obstet Gynecol* 1995;5:334–7

58. Schuchter K, Wald N, Hackshaw AK, Hafner E, Liebhart E. The distribution of nuchal translucency at 10–13 weeks of pregnancy. *Prenat Diagn* 1998;18:281–6

59. Pajkrt E, de Graaf IM, Mol BW, van Lith JM, Bleker OP, Bilardo CM. Weekly nuchal translucency measurements in normal fetuses. *Obstet Gynecol* 1998;91:208–11

60. Bernardino F, Cardoso R, Montenegro N, Bernardes J, de Sa JM. Semiautomated ultrasonographic measurement of fetal nuchal translucency using a computer software tool. *Ultrasound Med Biol* 1998; 24:51–4

61. Pandya PP, Snijders RJM, Johnson SJ, Brizot M, Nicolaides KH. Screening for fetal trisomies by maternal age and fetal nuchal translucency thickness at 10 to 14 weeks of gestation. *Br J Obstet Gynaecol* 1995;102:957–62

62. Snijders RJM, Noble P, Sebire N, Souka A, Nicolaides KH. UK multicentre project on assessment of risk of trisomy 21 by maternal age and fetal nuchal translucency thickness at 10–14 weeks of gestation. *Lancet* 1998;351:343–6

63. Johnson MP, Johnson A, Holzgreve W, Isada NB, Wapner RJ, Treadwell MC, Heeger S, Evans M. First-trimester simple hygroma: cause and outcome. *Am J Obstet Gynecol* 1993;168:156–61

64. Hewitt B. Nuchal translucency in the first trimester. *Aust NZ J Obstet Gynaecol* 1993;33:389–91

65. Shulman LP, Emerson D, Felker R, Phillips O, Simpson J, Elias S. High frequency of cytogenetic abnormalities with cystic hygroma diagnosed in the first trimester. *Obstet Gynecol* 1992;80:80–2

66. Nicolaides KH, Azar G, Byrne D, Mansur C, Marks K. Fetal nuchal translucency: ultrasound screening for chromosomal defects in first trimester of pregnancy. *Br Med J* 1992;304:867–89

67. Pandya PP, Kondylios A, Hilbert L, Snijders RJM, Nicolaides KH. Chromosomal defects and outcome in 1,015 fetuses with increased nuchal translucency. *Ultrasound Obstet Gynecol* 1995;5:15–19

68. Szabo J, Gellen J. Nuchal fluid accumulation in trisomy-21 detected by vaginal sonography in first trimester. *Lancet* 1990;336:1133

69. Wilson RD, Venir N, Faquharson DF. Fetal nuchal fluid – physiological or pathological? – in pregnancies less than 17 menstrual weeks. *Prenat Diagn* 1992;12:755–63

70. Ville Y, Lalondrelle C, Doumerc S, Daffos F, Frydman R, Oury JF, Dumez Y. First-trimester diagnosis of nuchal anomalies: significance and fetal outcome. *Ultrasound Obstet Gynecol* 1992;2:314–16

71. Trauffer ML, Anderson CE, Johnson A, Heeger S, Morgan P, Wapner RJ. The natural history of euploid pregnancies with first-trimester cystic hygromas. *Am J Obstet Gynecol* 1994;170:1279–84

72. Brambati B, Cislaghi C, Tului L, Alberti E, Amidani M, Colombo U, Zuliani G. First-trimester Down's syndrome screening using nuchal translucency: a prospective study. *Ultrasound Obstet Gynecol* 1995;5: 9–14

73. Comas C, Martinez JM, Ojuel J, Casals E, Puerto B, Borrell A, Fortuny A. First-trimester nuchal edema as a marker of aneuploidy. *Ultrasound Obstet Gynecol* 1995;5:26–9

74. Szabo J, Gellen J, Szemere G. First-trimester ultrasound screening for fetal aneuploidies in women over 35 and under 35 years of age. *Ultrasound Obstet Gynecol* 1995;5:161–3

75. Nadel A, Bromley B, Benacerraf BR. Nuchal thickening or cystic hygromas in first- and early second-trimester fetuses: prognosis and outcome. *Obstet Gynecol* 1993;82: 43–8

76. Savoldelli G, Binkert F, Achermann J, Schmid W. Ultrasound screening for chromosomal anomalies in the first trimester of pregnancy. *Prenat Diagn* 1993;13:513–18

77. Schulte-Vallentin M, Schindler H. Non-echogenic nuchal oedema as a marker in trisomy 21 screening. *Lancet* 1992;339:1053

78. Van Zalen-Sprock MM, Van Vugt JMG, Van Geijn HP. First-trimester diagnosis of cystic hygroma – course and outcome. *Am J Obstet Gynecol* 1992;167; 94–8

79. Cullen MT, Gabrielli S, Green JJ, Rizzo N, Mahoney MJ, Salafia C, Bovicelli L, Hobbins JC. Diagnosis and significance of cystic hygroma in the first trimester. *Prenat Diagn* 1990;10: 643–51

80. Suchet IB, Van der Westhuizen NG, Labatte MF. Fetal cystic hygromas: further insights into their natural history. *Can Assoc Radiol J* 1992;6:420–4

81. Pandya PP, Brizot ML, Kuhn P, Snijders RJM, Nicolaides KH. First trimester fetal nuchal translucency thickness and risk for trisomies. *Obstet Gynecol* 1994;84:420–3

82. Pandya PP, Goldberg H, Walton B, Riddle A, Shelley S, Snijders RJM, Nicolaides KH. The implementation of first-trimester scanning at 10–13 weeks' gestation and the measurement of fetal nuchal translucency thickness in two maternity units. *Ultrasound Obstet Gynecol* 1995;5:20–5

83. Bewley S, Roberts LJ, Mackinson M, Rodeck C. First trimester fetal nuchal translucency: problems with screening the general population. II. *Br J Obstet Gynaecol* 1995;102:386–8

84. Kornman LH, Morssink LP, Beekhuis JR, DeWolf BTHM, Heringa MP, Mantingh A. Nuchal translucency cannot be used as a screening test for chromosomal abnormalities in the first trimester of pregnancy in a routine ultrasound practice. *Prenat Diagn* 1996;16:797–805

85. Zimmerman R, Hucha A, Salvoldelli G, Binkert F, Acherman J, Grudzinskas JG. Serum parameters and nuchal translucency in first trimester screening for fetal chromosomal abnormalities. *Br J Obstet Gynaecol* 1996;103:1009–14

86. Taipale P, Hiilesmaa V, Salonen R, Ylostalo P. Increased nuchal translucency as a marker for fetal chromosomal defects. *N Engl J Med* 1997;337:1654–8

87. Hafner E, Schuchter K, Liebhart E, Philipp K. Results of routine fetal nuchal translucency measurement at 10–13 weeks in 4,233 unselected pregnant women. *Prenat Diagn* 1998;18: 29–34

88. Pajkrt E, van Lith JMM, Mol BWJ, Bleker OP, Bilardo CM. Screening for Down's syndrome by fetal nuchal translucency measurement in a general obstetric population. *Ultrasound Obstet Gynecol* 1998;12:163–9

89. Economides DL, Whitlow BJ, Kadir R, Lazanakis M, Verdin SM. First trimester sonographic detection of chromosomal abnormalities in an unselected population. *Br J Obstet Gynaecol* 1998; 105:58–62

90. Thilaganathan B, Slack A, Wathen NC. Effect of first-trimester nuchal translucency on second-trimester maternal serum biochemical screening for Down's syndrome. *Ultrasound Obstet Gynecol* 1997;10:261–4

91. Theodoropoulos P, Lolis D, Papageorgiou C, Papaioannou S, Plachouras N, Makrydimas G. Evaluation of first-trimester screening by fetal nuchal translucency and maternal age. *Prenat Diagn* 1998;18:133–7

92. Biagiotti R, Periti E, Brizzi L, Vanzi E, Cariati E. Comparison between two methods of standardization for gestational age differences in fetal nuchal translucency measurement in first-trimester screening for trisomy 21. *Ultrasound Obstet Gynecol* 1997;9:248–52

93. Orlandi F, Damiani G, Hallahan TW, Krantz DA, Macri JN. First-trimester screening for fetal aneuploidy: biochemistry and nuchal translucency. *Ultrasound Obstet Gynecol* 1997;10:381–6

94. Pandya PP, Snijders RJM, Johnson S, Nicolaides KH. Natural history of trisomy 21 fetuses with fetal nuchal translucency. *Ultrasound Obstet Gynecol* 1995;5:381–3

95. Hyett JH, Sebire NJ, Snijders RJM, Nicolaides KH. Intrauterine lethality of trisomy 21 fetuses with increased nuchal translucency. *Ultrasound Obstet Gynecol* 1996;7:101–3

96. Sherrod C, Sebire NJ, Soares W, Snijders RJ, Nicolaides KH. Prenatal diagnosis of trisomy 18 at the 10–14-week ultrasound scan. *Ultrasound Obstet Gynecol* 1997;10:387–90

97. Snijders RJM, Sebire NJ, Nayar R, Souka A, Nicolaides KH. Increased nuchal translucency in trisomy 13 fetuses at 10–14 weeks of gestation. *Am J Med Genet* 1999:in press

98. Sebire NJ, Snijders RJ, Brown R, Southall T, Nicolaides KH. Detection of sex chromosome abnormalities by nuchal translucency screening at 10–14 weeks. *Prenat Diagn* 1998;18:581–4

99. Jauniaux E, Brown R, Snijders RJ, Noble P, Nicolaides KH. Early prenatal diagnosis of triploidy. *Am J Obstet Gynecol* 1997;176:550–4

100. Reisman IE. Chromosomal abnormalities and intrauterine growth retardation. *Pediatr Clin North Am* 1970;17:101–10

101. Chen ATL, Chan YK, Falek A. The effects of chromosomal abnormalities on birth weight in man. *Hum Hered* 1972;22:209–24

102. Snijders RJ, Sherrod C, Gosden CM, Nicolaides KH. Fetal growth retardation: associated malformations and chromosomal abnormalities. *Am J Obstet Gynecol* 1993;168:547–55

103. Lynch L, Berkowitz RL. First trimester growth delay in trisomy 18. *Am J Perinatol* 1989;6:237–9

104. Drugan A, Johnson MP, Isada NB, Holzgreve W. Zador IE, Dombrowski MP, Sokol RJ, Hallak M, Evans MI. The smaller than expected first-trimester fetus is at increased risk for chromosome anomalies. *Am J Obstet Gynecol* 1992;167:1525–8

105. Kuhn P, Brizot ML, Pandya PP, Snijders RJ, Nicolaides KH. Crown-rump length in chromosomally abnormal fetuses at 10 to 13 weeks' gestation. *Am J Obstet Gynecol* 1995;172:32–5

106. Macintosh MC, Brambati B, Chard T, Grudzinskas JG. Crown–rump length in aneuploid fetuses: implications for first-trimester biochemical screening for aneuploidies. *Prenat Diagn* 1995;15:691–4

107. Bahado-Singh RO, Lynch L, Deren O, Morotti R, Copel J, Mahoney MJ, Williams J. First-trimester growth restriction and fetal aneuploidy: the effect of type of aneuploidy and gestational age. *Am J Obstet Gynecol* 1997;176:976–80

108. Schemmer G, Wapner RJ, Johnson A, Schemmer M, Norton HJ, Anderson WE. First-trimester growth patterns of aneuploid fetuses. *Prenat Diagn* 1997;17:155–9

109. Campbell S, Warsof SL, Little D, Cooper DJ. Routine ultrasound screening for the prediction of gestational age. *Obstet Gynecol* 1985;65:613–20

110. Bergsiø P, Denman III DW, Hoffman J, Meirik O. Duration of human singleton pregnancy. *Acta Obstet Gynecol Scand* 1990;69:197–207

111. Geirsson RT. Ultrasound instead of last menstrual period as the basis of gestational age assignment. *Ultrasound Obstet Gynecol* 1991;1:212–19

112. Schats R, Jansen CAM, Wladimiroff JW. Abnormal embryonic heart rate pattern in early pregnancy associated with Down's syndrome. *Hum Reprod* 1990;5: 877–9

113. Van Lith JMM, Visser GHA, Mantingh A, Beekhuis JR. Fetal heart rate in early pregnancy and chromosomal disorders. *Br J Obstet Gynaecol* 1992;99:741–4

114. Martinez JM, Echevarria M, Borrell A Puerto B, Ojuel J, Fortuny A. Fetal heart rate and nuchal translucency in detecting chromosomal abnormalities other than Down syndrome. *Obstet Gynecol* 1998;92:68–71

115. Hyett JA, Noble PL, Snijders RJ, Montenegro N, Nicolaides KH. Fetal heart rate in trisomy 21 and other chromosomal abnormalities at 10–14 weeks of gestation. *Ultrasound Obstet Gynecol* 1996;7: 239–44

116. Robinson HP, Shaw-Dunn J. Fetal heart rates as determined by sonar in early pregnancy. *J Obstet Gynaecol Br Commonw* 1973;90:805–9

117. Rempen A. Diagnosis of viability in early pregnancy with vaginal sonography. *J Ultrasound Med* 1990; 9:711–16

118. Wisser J, Dirschedl P. Embryonic heart rate in dated human embryos. *Early Hum Dev* 1994;37: 107–15

119. Wladimiroff JW, Seelen JC. Fetal heart action in early pregnancy. Development of fetal vagal function. *Eur J Obstet Gynecol* 1972;2:55–63

120. Hyett JA, Brizot ML, Von-Kaisenberg CS, McKie AT, Farzaneh F, Nicolaides KH. Cardiac gene expression of atrial natriuretic peptide and brain natriuretic peptide in trisomic fetuses. *Obstet Gynecol* 1996;87:506–10

121. Teitel D, Rudolph AM. Perinatal oxygen delivery and cardiac function. *Adv Paediatr* 1985;32: 321–47

122. Rudolph AM, Heymann MA. Cardiac output in the fetal lamb: the effects of spontaneous and induced changes of heart rate on right and left ventricular output. *Am J Obstet Gynecol* 1976;124: 183–92

123. Wladimiroff J, Huisman T, Stewart P. Fetal and umbilical blood flow velocity waveforms between 10 and 16 weeks gestation: a preliminary study. *Obstet Gynecol* 1991;78:812–14

124. Brown R, Di Luzio L, Gomes C, Nicolaides KH. The umbilical artery pulsatility index in the first trimester: is there an association with increased nuchal translucency or chromosomal abnormality? *Ultrasound Obstet Gynecol* 1998;12:244–7

125. Jauniaux E, Jurkovic D, Campbell S. *In vivo* investigation of the placental circulation by Doppler echography. *Placenta* 1995;16:323–31

126. Martinez JM, Borrell A, Antonin E, Puerto B, Casals E, Ojuel J, Fortuny A. Combining nuchal translucency and umbilical Doppler velocimetry for detecting fetal trisomies in the first trimester of pregnancy. *Br J Obstet Gynaecol* 1997;104:11–14

127. Jauniaux E, Gavrill P, Khun P, Kurdi W, Hyett J, Nicolaides KH. Fetal heart rate and umbilico-placental Doppler flow velocity waveforms in early pregnancies with a chromosomal abnormality and/or an increased nuchal translucency thickness. *Hum Reprod* 1996;11:435–9

128. Gudmundsson S, Huhta JC, Wood DC, Tulzer G, Cohen AW, Weiner S. Venous Doppler ultrasonography in the fetus with nonimmune hydrops. *Am J Obstet Gynecol* 1991;164:333–7

129. Reed KL, Appleton CP, Anderson CF, Shenker L, Sahn DJ. Doppler studies of vena cava flows in human fetuses. Insights into normal and abnormal cardiac physiology. *Circulation* 1990;81: 498–505

130. Reuss ML, Rudolph AM, Dae MW. Phasic blood flow patterns in the superior and inferior venae cavae and umbilical vein of fetal sheep. *Am J Obstet Gynecol* 1983;145:70–8

131. Brown RN, Di Luzio L, Gomes C, Nicolaides KH. First trimester umbilical venous Doppler sonography in chromosomally normal and abnormal fetuses. *J Ultrasound Med* 1999;18:543–6

132. Kiserud T. In a different vein: the ductus venosus could yield much valuable information. *Ultrasound Obstet Gynecol* 1997;9:369–72

133. Montenegro N, Matias A, Areias JC, Castedo S, Barros H. Increased fetal nuchal translucency: possible involvement of early cardiac failure. *Ultrasound Obstet Gynecol* 1997;10:265–8

134. Matias A, Gomes C, Flack N, Montenegro N, Nicolaides KH. Screening for chromosomal abnormalities at 11–14 weeks: the role of ductus venosus blood flow. *Ultrasound Obstet Gynecol* 1998;12:380–4

135. Brizot ML, Bersinger NA, Zydias G, Snijders RJ, Nicolaides KH. Maternal serum Schwangerschafts protein-1 (SP1) and fetal chromosomal abnormalities at 10–13 weeks of gestation. *Early Hum Dev* 1995;30:31–6

136. Brizot ML, Kuhn P, Bersinger NA, Snijders RJM, Nicolaides KH. First trimester maternal serum alpha-fetoprotein in fetal trisomies. *Br J Obstet Gynaecol* 1995;102:31–4

137. Noble PL, Wallace EM, Snijders RJM, Groome NP, Nicolaides KH. Maternal serum inhibin-A and free beta hCG concentrations in trisomy 21 pregnancies at 10–14 weeks of gestation. *Br J Obstet Gynaecol* 1997;104:367–71

138. Ozturk M, Milunsky A, Brambati B, Sachs ES, Miller SL, Wands JR. Abnormal maternal levels of hCG subunits in trisomy 18. *Am J Med Genet* 1990;36:480–3

139. Spencer K, Macri JN, Aitken DA, Connor JM. Free beta hCG as a first trimester marker for fetal trisomy. *Lancet* 1992;339:1480

140. Isles RK, Sharma K, Wathen NC, *et al.* hCG, free subunit and PAPP-A composition in normal and Down's syndrome pregnancies. In *Fourth conference: Endocrinology and Metabolism in Human Reproduction.* London: RCOG, 1993

141. Macri JN, Spencer K, Aitken DA, Garver K, Buchanan PD, Muller F, Boue A. First trimester free beta-hCG screening for Down syndrome. *Prenat Diagn* 1993;13:557–62

142. Pescia G, Marguerat PH, Weihs D, The HN, Maillard C, Loertscher A, Senn A. First trimester free beta-hCG and SP1 as markers for fetal chromosomal disorders: a prospective study of 250 women undergoing CVS. In *Fourth Conference: Endocrinology and Metabolism in Human Reproduction.* London: RCOG, 1993:45

143. Brambati B, Tului L, Bonacchi I, Shrimanker K, Suzuki Y, Grudzinskas JG. Serum PAPP-A and free beta hCG are first-trimester screening markers for Down syndrome. *Prenat Diagn* 1994;14:1043–7

144. Kellner LH, Weiss RR, Weiner Z, Neur M, Martin G. Early first trimester serum AFP, UE3, hCG and free beta-hCG measurements in unaffected and affected pregnancies with fetal Down syndrome. *Am J Hum Genet* 1994;55:A281

145. Forest J-C, Masse J, Moutquin J-M. Screening for Down syndrome during the first trimester: a prospective study using free b-human chorionic gonadotropin and pregnancy associated plasma protein-A. *Clin Biochem* 1997;30:333–8

146. Macintosh MCM, Iles R, Teisner B, Sharma K, Chard T, Grudzinskas JG, Ward RHT, Muller F. Maternal serum human chorionic gonadotrophin and pregnancy associated plasma protein A, markers for fetal Down syndrome at 8–14 weeks. *Prenat Diagn* 1994;14:203–8

147. Biagiotti R, Cariati E, Brizzi L, D'Agata A. Maternal serum screening for Down syndrome in the first trimester of pregnancy. *Br J Obstet Gynaecol* 1995;102: 660–2

148. Brizot ML, Snijders RJM, Butler J, Bersinger NA, Nicolaides KH. Maternal serum hCG and fetal nuchal translucency thickness for the prediction of fetal trisomies in the first trimester of pregnancy. *Br J Obstet Gynaecol* 1995;102:127–32

149. Noble PL, Abraha HD, Snijders RJM, Sherwood R, Nicolaides KH. Screening for fetal trisomy 21 in the first trimester of pregnancy: maternal serum free b–hCG and fetal nuchal translucency thickness. *Ultrasound Obstet Gynecol* 1996;6:390–5

150. Krantz DA, Larsen JW, Buchanan PD, Macri JN. First trimester Down syndrome screening: free β human chorionic gonadotropin and pregnancy associated plasma protein A. *Am J Obstet Gynecol* 1996;174:612–16

151. Scott F, Wheeler D, Sinosich M, Boogert A, Anderson J, Edelman D. First trimester aneuploidy screening using nuchal translucency, free beta human chorionic gonadotrophin and maternal age. *Aust NZ Obstet Gynaecol* 1996;36:381–4

152. Wald NJ, George L, Smith D, Densem JW, Petterson K, on behalf of the International Prenatal Screening Research Group. Serum screening for Down's syndrome between 8 and 14 weeks of pregnancy. *Br J Obstet Gynaecol* 1996;104:407–12

153. Berry E, Aitken DA, Crossley JA, Macri JN, Connor JM. Screening for Down's syndrome: changes in marker levels and detection rates between first and second trimester. *Br J Obstet Gynaecol* 1997; 104:811–17

154. Spencer K, Noble P, Snijders RJM, Nicolaides KH. First trimester urine free beta hCG, beta core and total oestriol in pregnancies affected by Down's syndrome: implications for first trimester screening with nuchal translucency and serum free beta hCG. *Prenat Diagn* 1997;17:525–38

155. Haddow JE, Palomaki GE, Knight GJ, Williams J, Miller WA, Johnson A. Screening of maternal serum for fetal Down's syndrome in the first trimester. *N Engl J Med* 1998;338:955–61

156. Wheeler DM, Sinosich MJ. Prenatal screening in the first trimester of pregnancy. *Prenat Diagn* 1998;18: 537–43

157. de Graaf IM, Pajkrt E, Bilardo CM, Leschot NJ, Cuckle HS, Van Lith JM. Early pregnancy screening for fetal aneuploidy with serum markers and nuchal translucency. *Prenat Diagn* 1999;19: 458–62

158. Spencer K, Souter V, Tul N, Snijders R, Nicolaides KH. A screening program for trisomy 21 at 10–14 weeks using fetal nuchal translucency, maternal serum free β–human chorionic gonadotropin and pregnancy-associated plasma protein-A. *Ultrasound Obstet Gynecol* 1999;13:231–7

159. Wald N, Stone R, Cuckle HS, Grudzinskas JG, Barkai G, Brambati B, Teisner B, Fuhrmann W. First trimester concentrations of pregnancy associated plasma protein A and placental protein 14 in Down's syndrome. *Br Med J* 1992;305:28

160. Brambati B, Macintosh MCM, Teisner B, Maguiness S, Shrimanker K, Lanzani A, Bonacchi I, Tului L, Chard T, Grudzinskas JG. Low maternal serum levels of pregnancy associated plasma protein A (PAPP-A) in the first trimester in association with abnormal fetal karyotype. *Br J Obstet Gynaecol* 1993;100:324–6

161. Hurley PA, Ward RHT, Teisner B, Isles RK, Lucas M, Grudzinskas JG. Serum PAPP-A measurements in first trimester screening for Down's syndrome. *Prenat Diagn* 1996;13:903–8

162. Muller F, Cuckle HS, Teisner B, Grudzinskas JG. Serum PAPP-A levels are depressed in women with fetal Down's syndrome in early pregnancy. *Prenat Diagn* 1993;13:633–6

163. Bersinger NA, Brizot ML, Johnson A, Snijders RJM, Abbott J, Schneider H, Nicolaides KH. First trimester maternal serum pregnancy-associated plasma protein A and pregnancy-specific β1-glycoprotein in fetal trisomies. *Br J Obstet Gynaecol* 1994;101:970–4

164. Brizot ML, Snijders RJM, Bersinger NA, Kuhn P, Nicolaides KH. Maternal serum pregnancy associated placental protein A and fetal nuchal translucency thickness for the prediction of fetal trisomies in early pregnancy. *Obstet Gynecol* 1994;84:918–22

165. Spencer K, Aitken DA, Crossley JA, McGaw G, Berry E, Anderson R, Connor JM, Macri JN. First trimester biochemical screening for trisomy 21: the role of free beta hCG, alpha fetoprotein and pregnancy associated plasma protein A. *Ann Clin Biochem* 1994;31:447–54

166. Casals E, Fortuny A, Grudzinskas JG, Suzuki Y, Teisner B, Comas C, Sanllehy C, Ojuel J, Borrell A, Soler A, Ballesta AM. First trimester biochemical screening for Down syndrome with the use of PAPP-A, AFP and β-hCG. *Prenat Diagn* 1996;16:405–10

167. Orlandi F, Damiani G, Hallahan TW, Krantz DA, Macri JN. First trimester screening for aneuploidy: biochemistry and nuchal translucency. *Ultrasound Obstet Gynecol* 1997;10:381–6

168. Tsukerman GL, Gusina NB, Cuckle HS. Maternal serum screening for Down syndrome in the first trimester: experience from Belarus. *Prenat Diagn* 1999;19:499–504

169. De Biasio P, Siccardi M, Volpe G, Famularo L, Santi P, Canini S. First trimester screening for Down's syndrome using nuchal translucency measurement with free β-hCG and PAPP-A between 10 and 13 weeks of pregnancy: the combined test. *Prenat Diagn* 1999;19:360–3

170. Wald NJ, Watt HC, Hackshaw AK. Integrated screening for Down's syndrome based on tests performed during the first and second trimesters. *N Engl J Med* 1999;341:461–7

171. Copel J, Bahado-Singh RO. Prenatal screening for Down's syndrome – a search for the family's values. *N Engl J Med* 1999;341:521–2

172. Kadir RA, Economides DL. The effect of nuchal translucency measurement on second trimester biochemical screening for Down's syndrome. *Ultrasound Obstet Gynecol* 1997;9:244–7

173. Thilaganathan B, Slack A, Wathen NC. Effect of first-trimester nuchal translucency on second-trimester maternal serum biochemical screening for Down's syndrome. *Ultrasound Obstet Gynecol* 1997;10:261–4

174. Nicolaides KH, Snijders RJM, Gosden CM, Berry C, Campbell S. Ultrasonographically detectable markers of fetal chromosomal abnormalities. *Lancet* 1992;340:704–7

175. Snijders RJM, Nicolaides KH. Assessment of risks. In *Ultrasound Markers for Fetal Chromosomal Defects*. Carnforth, UK: Parthenon Publishing, 1996:63–120

176. Snijders RJ, Sebire NJ, Faria M, Patel F, Nicolaides KH. Fetal mild hydronephrosis and chromosomal defects: relation to maternal age and gestation. *Fetal Diagn Ther* 1995;10:349–55

177. Snijders RJM, Shawa L, Nicolaides KH. Fetal choroid plexus cysts and trisomy 18: assessment of risk based on ultrasound findings and maternal age. *Prenat Diagn* 1994;14:1119–27

178. Nyberg DA, Luthy DA, Resta RG, Nyberg BC, Williams MA. Age-adjusted ultrasound risk assessment for fetal Down's syndrome during the second trimester: description of the method and analysis of 142 cases. *Ultrasound Obstet Gynecol* 1998;12:8–14

179. Donnenfeld AE, Carlson DE, Palomaki GE, Librizzi RJ, Weiner S, Platt L. Prospective multicenter study of second trimester nuchal skinfold thickness in unaffected and Down syndrome pregnancies. *Obstet Gynecol* 1994;84:844–7

180. Biagiotti R, Periti E, Cariati E. Humerus and femur length in fetuses with Down syndrome. *Prenat Diagn* 1994;14:429–34

181. Cuckle H, Wald N, Quinn J, Royston P, Butler L. Ultrasound fetal femur length measurement in the screening for Down's syndrome. *Br J Obstet Gynaecol* 1989;96:1373–8

182. Grandjean H, Sarramon MF. Femur/foot length ratio for detection of Down syndrome: results of a multicenter prospective study. The Association Francaise pour le Depistage et la Prevention des Handicaps de l'Enfant Study Group. *Am J Obstet Gynecol* 1995;173:16–19

183. Johnson MP, Michaelson JE, Barr M, Treadwell MC, Hume RF, Dombrowski MP, Evans MI. Combining humerus and femur length for improved ultrasonographic identification of pregnancies at increased risk for trisomy 21. *Am J Obstet Gynecol* 1995;172:1229–35

184. Owen J, Wenstrom KD, Hardin JM, Boots LR, Hsu CC, Cosper PC, DuBard MB. The utility of fetal biometry as an adjunct to the multiple-marker screening test for Down syndrome. *Am J Obstet Gynecol* 1994;17:1041–6

185. Vintzileos AM, Egan JF, Smulian JC, Campbell WA, Guzman ER, Rodis JF. Adjusting the risk for trisomy 21 by a simple ultrasound method using fetal long-bone biometry. *Obstet Gynecol* 1996;87:953–8

186. Bromley B, Doubilet P, Frigoletto FD, Jr, Krauss C, Estroff JA, Benacerraf BR. Is fetal hyperechoic bowel on second-trimester sonogram an indication for amniocentesis? *Obstet Gynecol* 1994;83:647–51

187. Corteville JE, Gray DL, Langer JC. Bowel abnormalities in the fetus – correlation of prenatal ultrasonographic findings with outcome. *Am J Obstet Gynecol* 1996;175:724–9

188. Muller F, Dommergues M, Aubry MC, Simon-Bouy B, Gautier E, Oury JF, Narcy F. Hyperechogenic fetal bowel: an ultrasonographic marker for adverse fetal and neonatal outcome. *Am J Obstet Gynecol* 1995;173:508–13

189. Homola J. Are echogenic foci in fetal heart ventricles insignificant findings?. *Ceska Gynekologie* 1997;62:280–2

190. Simpson JM, Cook A, Sharland G. The significance of echogenic foci in the fetal heart: a prospective study of 228 cases. *Ultrasound Obstet Gynecol* 1996;8:225–8

191. Vibhakar NI, Budorick NE, Sciosia AL, Harby LD, Mullen ML, Sklansky MS. Prevalence of aneuploidy with a cardiac intraventricular echogenic focus in an at-risk patient population. *J Ultrasound Med* 1999;18:265–8

192. Vintzileos AM, Campbell WA, Guzman ER, Smulian JC, McLean DA, Ananth CV. Second-trimester ultrasound markers for detection of trisomy 21: which markers are best? *Obstet Gynecol* 1997;89:941–4

193. Wickstrom EA, Thangavelu M, Parilla BV, Tamura RK, Sabbagha RE. A prospective study of the association between isolated fetal pyelectasis and chromosomal abnormality. *Obstet Gynecol* 1996;88:379–82

194. Bianchi DW, Flint AF, Pizzimenti MF, Knoll JHM, Latt SA. Isolation of fetal DNA from nucleated erythrocytes in maternal blood. *Proc Natl Acad Sci USA* 1990;87:3279–83

195. Price JO, Elias S, Wachtel S, Klinger K, Dockter M, Tharapel A, Shulman LP, Phillips OP, Meyers CM, Shook D, Simpso JL. Prenatal diagnosis with fetal cells isolated from maternal blood by multiparameter flow cytometry. *Am J Obstet Gynecol* 1991;165:1731–7

196. Hamada H, Arinami T, Kubo T, Hamaguchi H, Iwasaki H. Fetal nucleated cells in maternal peripheral blood: frequency and relationship to gestational age. *Hum Genet* 1993;91:427–32

197. Ganshirt-Ahlert D, Burschyk M, Garritsen HSP, Helmer L, Miny P, Horst J, Schneider HPG, Holzgreve W. Magnetic cell sorting and the transferrin receptor as potential means of prenatal diagnosis from maternal blood. *Am J Obstet Gynecol* 1992;166:1350–5

198. Wachtel S, Elias S, Price J, Wachtel G, Phillips O, Shulman L, Meyers C, Simpson JL, Dockter M. Fetal cells in the maternal circulation: isolation by multiparameter flow cytometry and confirmation by polymerase chain reaction. *Hum Reprod* 1991;6:1466–9

199. Al-Mufti R, Hambley H, Farzaneh F, Nicolaides KH. Investigation of maternal blood enriched for fetal cells: Role in screening and diagnosis of fetal trisomies. *Am J Med Genet* 1999;85:66–75

200. Durrant LG, MeDowall KM, Holmes RA, Liu DTY. Screening of monoclonal antibodies recognizing oncofetal antigens for isolation of trophoblasts from maternal blood for prenatal diagnosis. *Prenat Diagn* 1994;14:131–40

201. Pandya PP, Kuhn P, Brizot M, Cardy DL, Nicolaides KH. Rapid detection of chromosome aneuploides in fetal blood and chorionic villi by fluorescence in situ hybridisation (FISH). *Br J Obstet Gynaecol* 1994;101:493–7

202. Bianchi DW, Mahr A, Zickwolf GK, House TW, Flint AF, Klinger KW. Detection of fetal cells with 47XY,+21 karyotype in maternal peripheral blood. *Hum Genet* 1992; 90:368–70

203. Ganshirt-Ahlert D, Borjesson-Stoll R, Burschyk M, Dohr A, Garritsen HSP, Helmer L, Miny P, Velasco M, Walde C, Patterson D, Teng N, Bhat NM, Bieber MM, Holzgreve W. Detection of fetal trisomies 21 and 18 from maternal blood using triple gradient and magnetic cell sorting. *Am J Reprod Immunol* 1993;30:194–201

204. Simpson JL, Elias S. Isolating fetal cells in maternal circulation for prenatal diagnosis. *Prenat Diagn* 1994;14:1229–42

205. Ager RP, Oliver RW. In *The Risks of Mid-trimester Amniocentesis, Being a Comparative, Analytical Review of the Major Clinical Studies*. Salford University, 1986

206. Tabor A, Philip J, Madsen M, Bang J, Obel EB, Norgaard-Pedersen B. Randomised controlled trial of genetic amniocentesis in 4,606 low-risk women. *Lancet* 1986;i:1287–93

207. Nicolaides KH, Brizot M, Patel F, Snijders R. Comparison of chorionic villus sampling and amniocentesis for fetal karyotyping at 10–13 weeks' gestation. *Lancet* 1994;344:435–9

208. Sundberg K, Bang J, Smidt-Jensen S, *et al*. Randomised study of risk of fetal loss related to early amniocentesis versus chorionic villus sampling. *Lancet* 1997;350:697–703

209. CEMAT Group. Randomised trial to assess safety and fetal outcome of early and mid-trimester amniocentesis. *Lancet* 1998;351:242–7

210. Canadian Collaborative CVS–Amniocentesis Clinical Trial Group. Multicentre randomised clinical trial of chorion villus sampling and amniocentesis. *Lancet* 1989;i:1–6

211. Smidt-Jensen S, Permin M, Philip J, Lundsteen C, Zachary JM, Fowler SE, Gruning K. Randomised comparison of amniocentesis and transabdominal and transcervical chorionic villus sampling. *Lancet* 1992;340:1238–44

212. Ammala P, Hiilesmaa VK, Liukkonen S, Saisto T, Teramo K, Von Koskull H. Randomized trial comparing first trimester transcervical chorionic villus sampling and second trimester amniocentesis. *Prenat Diagn* 1993;13:919–27

213. European study: MRC working party on the evaluation of chorion villus sampling. Medical Research Council European trial of chorion villus sampling. *Lancet* 1991;337:1491–9

214. Firth HV, Boyd PA, Chamberlain P, MacKenzie IZ, Lindenbaum RH, Huson SM. Severe limb abnormalities after chorion villous sampling at 56–66 days' gestation. *Lancet* 1991;337:762–3

215. Firth HV, Boyd PA, Chamberlain PF, MacKenzie IZ, Morriss-Kay GM, Huson SM. Analysis of limb reduction defects in babies exposed to chorion villus sampling. *Lancet* 1994;343:1069–71

216. Froster-Iskenius UG, Baird PA. Limb reduction defects in over one million consecutive livebirths. *Teratology* 1989;39:127–35

217. Foster UG, Jackson L. Limb defects and chorionic villus sampling; results from an international registry 1992–94. *Lancet* 1996;347:489–94

2

Increased nuchal translucency with normal karyotype

Increased fetal nuchal translucency thickness at 11–14 weeks of gestation is a common phenotypic expression of trisomy 21 and other chromosomal defects[1,2]. Extensive studies have now established that, in chromosomally normal fetuses, increased nuchal translucency is also associated with a wide range of fetal defects and genetic syndromes.

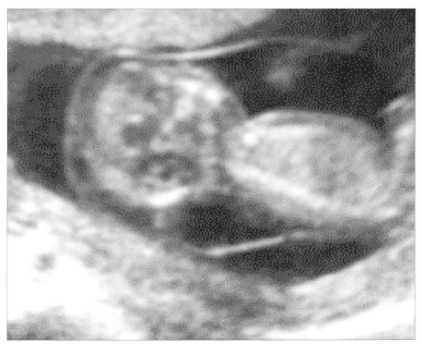

Figure 1   Massively increased nuchal translucency thickness in a 13-week chromosomally normal fetus

SMALL SERIES

In the combined data from several small series, on a total of 510 chromosomally normal fetuses with increased nuchal translucency, there were 77 (15%) with defects (Table 1)[3–21].

The most commonly seen defects were anencephaly ($n = 1$), macrocephaly ($n = 1$), spina bifida ($n = 2$), holoprosencephaly ($n = 1$), Dandy–Walker malformation ($n = 1$), facial cleft ($n = 2$), agnathia ($n = 1$), cystic hygromas ($n = 1$), cardiac defects ($n = 17$), pentalogy of Cantrell ($n = 1$), Ivemark syndrome ($n = 1$), Toriello–Carey syndrome ($n = 1$), diaphragmatic hernia ($n = 2$), esophageal atresia ($n = 1$), duodenal atresia ($n = 1$), exomphalos ($n = 4$), megacystis ($n = 3$), multicystic kidneys ($n = 1$), polycystic kidneys ($n = 3$), amnion rupture sequence ($n = 1$), body stalk anomaly ($n = 2$), achondrogenesis ($n = 1$), achondroplasia ($n = 2$), campomelic dysplasia ($n = 1$), ectrodactyly-ectodermal dysplasia–cleft palate syndrome (EEC) ($n = 1$), fetal akinesia deformation sequence (FADS) ($n = 3$), syringomyelia ($n = 1$), kyphosis ($n = 1$), talipes ($n = 1$), GM1-gangliosidosis ($n = 1$), Joubert syndrome ($n = 1$), Meckel–Gruber syndrome ($n = 1$), myotonic dystrophy ($n = 1$), Noonan syndrome ($n = 5$), spinal muscular atrophy ($n = 2$), Zellweger syndrome ($n = 1$) and unspecified syndromes ($n = 6$).

THE FETAL MEDICINE FOUNDATION PROJECT

In the multicenter screening project for trisomy 21 by a combination of maternal age and fetal nuchal translucency involving about 100 000 pregnancies[1], there were 4116 singleton, chromosomally normal pregnancies with fetal nuchal translucency above the 95th centile for crown–rump length[22]. This study includes data on the first 565 cases reported by Pandya et al.[23] and those on 89 cases which had detailed postnatal follow up[24]. A wide range of structural defects and genetic syndromes were identified in 161(3.9%) of the cases (Table 2)[22].

The patients were subdivided according to nuchal translucency thickness into five groups: 95th centile to 3.4 mm, 3.5–4.4 mm, 4.5–5.4 mm, 5.5–6.4 and ≥ 6.5 mm. The prevalence of fetal abnormalities increased with nuchal translucency thickness: 3 mm, 2.4%; 4 mm, 7.1%; 5 mm, 12.3%; 6 mm, 16.7%; 7 mm 35.6% (Table 2)[22]. The diagnosis of abnormalities was made by ultrasound examination in mid-pregnancy, or by pathological examination in terminations of pregnancy and intrauterine or neonatal deaths, or by clinical examination and appropriate investigations in live births. In these calculations, we did not include minor defects, such as choroid plexus cysts, pyelectasia, digital abnormalities or cardiac defects that would not require therapy[22].

Table 1 Studies reporting defects in chromosomally normal fetuses with increased nuchal translucency (NT) thickness at 10–14 weeks of gestation. The cut-off of increased NT varied between the studies

Authors	NT	n		Other defects
Johnson et al. 1993[3] Trauffer et al. 1994[4]	> 2.0	32	5	megacystis (1), amnion rupture sequence (1), Noonan syndrome (1), unspecified syndrome (2)
Shulman et al. 1994[5]	≥ 2.5	32	1	cystic hygromas (1)
Hafner et al. 1998[6]	≥ 2.5	72	7	campomelic dysplasia (1), cardiac defect (2), exomphalos (1), pentalogy of Cantrell (1), Ivemark syndrome (1), Toriello–Carey syndrome (1)
van Zalen-Sprock et al. 1992[7]	≥ 3.0	13	3	megacystis (1), polycystic kidneys (1), Noonan syndrome (1)
Ville et al. 1992[8]	≥ 3.0	61	10	facial cleft (1), cardiac defects (3), multicystic kidneys (1), exomphalos (1), FADS (2), unspecified syndrome (2)
Hewitt 1993[9]	≥ 3.0	10	1	achondrogenesis (1)
Salvesen et al. 1995[10]	≥ 3.0	5	2	holoprosencephaly (1), cardiac defect (1)
Hewitt et al. 1996[11]	≥ 3.0	44	3	syringomyelia (1), body stalk anomaly (1), kyphosis (1)
Reynders et al. 1997[12]	≥ 3.0	35	3	polycystic kidneys (1), Noonan syndrome (1), Joubert syndrome (1)
Hernadi & Torocsik 1997[13]	≥ 3.0	17	2	achondroplasia (1), body stalk anomaly (1)
Bilardo et al. 1998[14]	≥ 3.0	47	11	Dandy–Walker malformation (1), agnathia (1), cardiac defects (2), EEC syndrome (1), esophageal atresia (1), Noonan syndrome (1), Zellweger syndrome (1), GM1-gangliosidosis (1), myotonic dystrophy (1), spinal muscular atrophy (1)
Pajkrt et al. 1998[15]	≥ 3.0	21	1	cardiac defect (1)
Van Vugt et al. 1998[16]	≥ 3.0	63	8	Meckel–Gruber (1), diaphragmatic hernia (1), cardiac defects (2), duodenal atresia (1), polycystic kidneys (1), megacystis (1), spinal muscular atrophy (1)
Nadell et al. 1993[17]	≥ 4.0	16	5	facial cleft (1), cardiac defects (1), diaphragmatic hernia (1), exomphalos (1), FADS (1)
Moselhi et al. 1996[18]	≥ 4.0	8	3	cardiac defects (2), spina bifida (1)
Thilaganathan et al. 1997[19] Adekunle et al. 1999[20]	≥ 4.0	30	10	anencephaly (1), spina bifida (1), cardiac defects (2), exomphalos (1), talipes (1), Noonan syndrome (1), macrocephaly (1), unspecified syndrome (2)
Fukada et al. 1998[21]	≥ 5.0	4	2	cardiac defect (1), achondroplasia (1)

FAD, fetal akinesia deformation sequence; EEC, ectrodactyly-ectodermal dysplasia-cleft palate syndrome

Table 2 Fetal defects and genetic syndromes identified in the 4116 pregnancies with increased fetal nuchal translucency in The Fetal Medicine Foundation Project[22]

Fetal abnormality	Fetal nuchal translucency thickness (mm)					Pregnancy outcome		
	< 3.5	3.5–4.4	4.5–5.4	5.5–6.4	≥ 6.5	TOP	Death	Alive
Anencephaly	4	1				5		
Encephalocoele	3a				1	4		
Ventriculomegaly	6					5		1
Dandy–Walker cyst	1					1		
Holoprosencephaly	1					1		
Microcephaly	1							1
Facial cleft	2							2
Microphthalmia	1b							1
Laryngeal cyst	1							1
Cystic hygroma	1							1
Major cardiac defect	12	12	6	3	10	19	9	15
Diaphragmatic hernia	4	1	3			1	5	2
Exomphalos	2c	3de	1f	1g		5	1	1
Gastroschisis		1					1	
Bowel obstruction	2							2
Duodenal atresia		1						1
Hydronephrosis	2	2	1			1		4
Multicystic kidneys	4					3		1b
Polycystic kindeys					1	1		
Renal agenesis	1	1				1		1b
Megacystis	7	1				2	2	4
Spina bifida	3	1				2	1	1
Kyphoscoliosis				1		1		
Body stalk anomaly	1	3	1	1	4	10		
Diastomatomelia	1							1
Talipes	10	4	1			1		14
Akinesia deformation	2			1	3	6		
Jarcho–Levin syndrome	1		1			1	1	
Joubert syndrome	1					1		
Nance–Sweeney syndrome			1					1
Noonan syndrome					1			1
Smith–Lemli–Opitz	1		1	1		2	1	
Spinal muscular atrophy	1						1	
Thanatophoric dysplasia	1					1		
Trigonocephaly 'C'	1							1
VACTERL association	2					1		1
Unspecified syndrome	3	1	1		1	2		4
Total	83 (2.4%)	32 (7.1%)	17 (12.3%)	8 (16.7%)	21 (35.6%)			

a, encephalocele + AVSD; b, unilateral; c, spina bifida + cloacal exstrophy; d, Beckwith-Wiedemann syndrome; e, extrocardia; f, spina bifida + anencephaly, g, spina bifida + coarctation of aorta

TOP, termination of pregnancy; AVSD, atrioventricular septal defect

Pregnancy outcome

In the 4116 pregnancies, there were 3885 live births that survived the neonatal period, 38 neonatal deaths, 74 spontaneous abortions or intrauterine deaths and 77 terminations at the request of the parents, because fetal abnormalities were detected by ultrasonography in the first trimester or at follow-up scans; termination of pregnancy was also performed in 42 cases because of the uncertain prognosis, since a repeat scan 2 weeks after presentation demonstrated persistence or increase in the large translucency (Table 3)[22].

Table 3 Outcome in 4116 pregnancies with increased fetal nuchal translucency in The Fetal Medicine Foundation Project[22]

Nuchal translucency (mm)	Total	Termination (abnormal)	Prenatal death	Postnatal death	Alive
95th–3.4	3423	49 (36)	47	29	3298 (96.3%)
3.5–4.4	448	23 (14)	9	4	412 (92.0%)
4.5–5.4	138	13 (8)	4	3	118 (85.5%)
5.5–6.4	48	13 (7)	4	0	31 (64.6%)
≥ 6.5	59	21 (12)	10	2	26 (44.4%)
Total	4116	119 (77)	74	38	3885 (94.4%)

FETAL DEFECTS PRESENTING WITH INCREASED NUCHAL TRANSLUCENCY THICKNESS

An increasing number of fetal abnormalities can now be diagnosed by ultrasound examination in early pregnancy. A review of the literature for studies reporting the diagnosis of fetal abnormalities at the 11–14-week scan identified several conditions that were associated with increased nuchal translucency thickness (Table 4)[25–57].

CONSEQUENCES OF INCREASED NUCHAL TRANSLUCENCY

Increased nuchal translucency at the 11–14-week scan is associated with a wide range of fetal abnormalities. The observed prevalence for some of the abnormalities, such as anencephaly, holoprosencephaly, microcephaly, facial cleft, gastroschisis, renal abnormalities, bowel obstruction and spina bifida, may not be different from that in the general population. However, the prevalence of major cardiac defects, diaphragmatic hernia, exomphalos, body stalk anomaly and fetal akinesia deformation sequence appears to be substantially higher than in the general population and it is therefore likely

Table 4 Case reports and series of fetal abnormalities diagnosed by early ultrasound examination and found to be associated with increased nuchal translucency thickness (NT)

Abnormality	Gestation (weeks)	Increased NT	Authors
Cardiac defect	10–14	17 of 21	Gembruch et al. 1990[25], 1993[26], Bronshtein et al. 1990[27], Achiron et al. 1994[28]
Diaphragmatic hernia	10–14	8 of 20	Sebire et al. 1998[29], Lam et al. 1998[30]
Exomphalos	11–14	8 of 14	van Zalen-Sprock et al. 1997[31]
Achondrogenesis type II	11–12	2 of 2	Fisk et al. 1991[32], Soothill et al. 1993[33]
Asphyxiating thoracic dystrophy	14	1 of 1	Ben Ami et al. 1997[34]
Blomstrand osteochondrodysplasia	12	1 of 1	den Hollander et al. 1997[35]
Body stalk anomaly	10–14	10 of 14	Daskalakis et al. 1997[36]
Ectrodactyly-ectodermal dysplasia	14	1 of 1	Leung et al. 1995[37]
Fetal akinesia deformation sequence	10–14	2 of 2	Hyett et al. 1997[38]
Fryn syndrome	12	2 of 2	Bulas 1992[39], Hosli et al. 1997[40]
Hydrolethalus syndrome	11–12	2 of 2	Ammala & Salonen 1995[41], de Ravel et al. 1999[42]
Jarcho–Levin syndrome	12	2 of 4	Eliyahu et al. 1997[43], Lam et al. 1999[44]
Meckel–Gruber syndrome	11	1 of 6	Quintero et al. 1993[45], Sepulveda et al. 1997[46]
Megacystis	10–14	6 of 15	Sebire et al. 1996[47]
Osteogenesis imperfecta II	11	2 of 2	Makrydimas et al. 1999[48]
Perlman syndrome	11	1 of 1	van der Stege et al. 1998[49]
Roberts syndrome	11	1 of 1	Petrikovsky et al. 1997[50]
Short-rib polydactyly syndrome I	13	1 of 1	Hill & Leary 1998[51]
Smith–Lemli–Opitz syndrome	10–11	3 of 3	Hobbins et al. 1994[52], Hyett et al. 1995[53], Sharp et al. 1997[54]
Spinal muscular atrophy I	11–13	2 of 2	Rijhsinghani et al. 1997[55], Stiller et al. 1999[56]
Zellweger syndrome	12	1 of 1	de Graaf et al. 1999[57]

that there is an association between these abnormalities and increased nuchal translucency thickness. Similarly, there may well be an association between increased translucency and a wide range of rare skeletal dysplasias and genetic syndromes that are usually found in less than 1 in 10 000 pregnancies; however, the number of affected cases, both in the present and previous series of fetuses with increased nuchal translucency, is too small for definite conclusions to be drawn.

In addition to the association between increased nuchal translucency thickness and a wide range of fetal abnormalities, the rates of miscarriage and perinatal death increase with nuchal translucency thickness. These data would be useful in counselling parents of affected pregnancies and in alerting sonographers to plan the appropriate follow-up investigations for such pregnancies. However, it should be emphasized to the parents that increased nuchal translucency thickness *per se* does not constitute a fetal abnormality and, once chromosomal defects have been excluded, about 90% of pregnancies with fetal translucency below 4.5 mm would result in healthy live births; the rates for translucency of 4.5–6.4 mm and 6.5 mm or more are about 80% and 45%, respectively[22].

CONDITIONS ASSOCIATED WITH INCREASED NUCHAL TRANSLUCENCY

The fetal abnormalities and genetic syndromes associated with increased nuchal translucency are summarized in Table 5.

Table 5 Conditions associated with increased nuchal translucency

Cardiac defects	Jarcho–Levin syndrome
Diaphragmatic hernia	Joubert syndrome
Exomphalos	Meckel–Gruber syndrome
Achondrogenesis type II	Nance–Sweeney syndrome
Achondroplasia	Noonan syndrome
Asphyxiating thoracic dystrophy	Osteogenesis imperfecta type II
Beckwith–Wiedemann syndrome	Perlman syndrome
Blomstrand osteochondrodysplasia	Roberts syndrome
Body stalk anomaly	Short-rib polydactyly syndrome
Campomelic dysplasia	Smith–Lemli–Opitz syndrome
EEC syndrome	Spinal muscular atrophy type 1
Fetal akinesia deformation sequence	Thanatophoric dysplasia
Fryn syndrome	Trigonocephaly 'C' syndrome
GM1-gangliosidosis	VACTERL association
Hydrolethalus syndrome	Zellweger syndrome

EEC syndrome, ectrodactyly-ectodermal dysplasia-cleft palate syndrome

CARDIAC DEFECTS

Increased nuchal translucency is of particular importance in its association with major abnormalities of the heart and great arteries. Studies involving pathological examination in both chromosomally abnormal and normal fetuses with increased nuchal translucency at 11–14 weeks have demonstrated a high prevalence of abnormalities of the heart and great arteries[58–63]. Additionally, there are several case reports or small series on the sonographic diagnosis of cardiac defects at the 11–14-week scan; in a total of 21 fetuses with major cardiac defects, 17 (81%) had increased nuchal translucency[25–28]. Furthermore, a retrospective study of 1389 chromosomally normal fetuses with increased translucency reported that the prevalence of major cardiac defects increased with translucency thickness; the diagnosis of cardiac defects was made by ultrasound examination in mid-pregnancy, or by pathological examination in terminations of pregnancy and intrauterine or neonatal deaths, or by clinical examination and appropriate investigations in livebirths[63].

In The Fetal Medicine Foundation Project (Table 2, p. 70), the prevalence of major abnormalities of the heart and great arteries was 10 per 1000 and increased exponentially with increasing translucency thickness from about 4 per 1000 for translucency of 95th centile–3.4 mm, 27 per 1000 for translucency of 3.5–4.4 mm, 43 per 1000 for translucency of 4.5–5.4 mm, 63 per 1000 for translucency of 5.5–6.4 mm, and 169 per 1000 for translucency of ≥ 6.5 mm[22].

A retrospective study of 29 154 chromosomally normal singleton pregnancies identified major defects of the heart and great arteries in 50 cases (these included 18 that were diagnosed antenatally by an ultrasound examination at 16–31 weeks of gestation, 13 that were diagnosed at pathological examination following intrauterine death or termination of pregnancy for conditions other than cardiac defects, and 19 that were diagnosed in live births)[64]. The prevalence of major cardiac defects increased with nuchal translucency thickness from 0.8 per 1000 for those with translucency below the 95th centile to 63.5 per 1000 for translucency above the 99th centile (Table 6)[64].

Table 6 Prevalence of major defects of the heart and great arteries in chromosomally normal fetuses by nuchal translucency thickness[64]

Nuchal translucency (mm)	n	Major cardiac defects	Prevalence (per 1000)
< 95th centile	27 332	22	0.8
≥ 95th centile–3.4	1 507	8	5.3
3.5–4.4	208	6	28.9
4.5–5.4	66	6	90.9
≥ 5.5	41	8	195.1
Total	29 154	50	1.7

The distribution of different types of cardiac defects was similar to that described in previous prenatal and postnatal series (Table 7)[64]. Although increased nuchal translucency was observed with all types of major abnormalities of the heart and great arteries, there was a stronger association with left-sided defects, such as hypoplastic left heart and coarctation of the aorta. The sensitivity, specificity, positive and negative predictive values of nuchal translucency thickness cut-offs of the 95th and 99th centiles

Table 7 Detection of specific cardiac defects using increased fetal nuchal translucency thickness[64]

Cardiac defect	Total	Nuchal translucency	
		> 95th centile	> 99th centile
Tetralogy of Fallot	9 (18%)	2 (22%)	2 (22%)
Hypoplastic left heart	3 (6%)	2 (67%)	1 (33%)
Transposition of the great arteries	8 (16%)	4 (50%)	3 (38%)
Coarctation of the aorta or aortic stenosis/atresia	10 (20%)	10 (100%)	8 (80%)
Ventricular and atrioventricular septal defects	8 (16%)	4 (50%)	1 (13%)
Other defects	12 (24%)	6 (50%)	5 (42%)
Total	50 (100%)	28 (56%)	20 (40%)

Table 8 Sensitivity and specificity of screening for major defects of the heart and great arteries using fetal nuchal translucency[64]

	Using 95th centile	Using 99th centile
Sensitivity	56.0% (95% CI: 42.0–70.0)	40.0% (95% CI: 26.0–54.0)
Specificity	93.8% (95% CI: 93.6–94.1)	99.0% (95% CI: 98.9–99.1)
Positive predictive value	1.5% (95% CI: 1.0–2.1)	6.3% (95% CI: 3.7–9.0)
Negative predictive value	99.9% (95% CI: 99.8–100.0)	99.9% (95% CI: 99.8–100.0)

CI, confidence interval

in the detection of major cardiac defects are shown in Table 8; essentially 40% of all cardiac defects were in the subgroup with translucency above the 99th centile, and 56% were in the subgroup with translucency above the 95th centile[64].

In a prospective study of 398 chromosomally normal fetuses with a nuchal translucency measurement above the 99th centile (≥ 3.5 mm), specialist fetal echocardiography was carried out[65]. Major cardiac defects were present in 29 (7.6%) cases and, in 28 of these, the diagnosis was made by antenatal echocardiography. The prevalence of cardiac defects increased from 3% in those with a nuchal translucency of 3.5–5.4 mm to 15% in those with a measurement of 5.5 mm or more.

The clinical implication of these findings is that increased nuchal translucency constitutes an indication for specialist fetal echocardiography. Certainly, the overall prevalence of major cardiac defects in such a group of fetuses (about 2%) is similar to that found in pregnancies affected by maternal diabetes mellitus or with a history of a previously affected offspring, which are well accepted indications for fetal echocardiography. At present, there may not be sufficient facilities for specialist fetal echocardiography to accommodate the potential increase in demand if the 95th centile of nuchal translucency thickness is used as the cut-off for referral. In contrast, a cut-off of the 99th centile would result in only a small increase in workload and, in this population, the prevalence of major cardiac defects would be very high (about 6%).

Patients identified by nuchal translucency scanning as being at high risk for cardiac defects need not wait until 20 weeks for specialist echocardiography. Improvements in the resolution of ultrasound machines have now made it possible to undertake detailed cardiac scanning in the first trimester of pregnancy[26,65–68]. A specialist scan from 14 weeks can effectively reassure the majority of parents that there is no major cardiac defect. In the cases with a major defect, the early scan can either lead to the correct diagnosis or at least raise suspicions so that follow-up scans are carried out.

DIAPHRAGMATIC HERNIA

This is a sporadic defect with a birth prevalence of about 1 in 4000. In about 50% of affected fetuses, there are associated chromosomal abnormalities or other defects. In those with isolated diaphragmatic hernia, survival after postnatal surgery is about 50%, but the remainder die due to pulmonary hypoplasia and pulmonary hypertension[69].

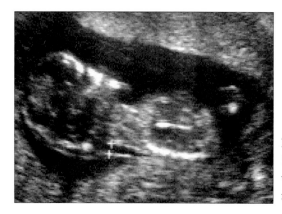

Figure 2 Stomach in the chest of a 13-week chromosomally normal fetus with diaphragmatic hernia and increasing nuchal translucency thickness

In The Fetal Medicine Foundation Project, the prevalence of diaphragmatic hernia (eight in 4116)[22], was higher than expected in the general population, suggesting an association between this defect and increased nuchal translucency. This was indeed found to be the case in a multicenter ultrasound screening study for chromosomal defects by a combination of maternal age and fetal nuchal translucency[29]. In a total of

78 639 pregnancies presumed to be normal chromosomally, there were 19 cases with diaphragmatic hernia, which was diagnosed at the initial or subsequent scans or at birth. At the early scan, the nuchal translucency was increased in 37% of cases of diaphragmatic hernia, including 83% of those that resulted in neonatal death due to pulmonary hypoplasia and in 22% of the survivors[29]. See Chapter 3 for the pathophysiology of increased nuchal translucency in diaphragmatic hernia.

EXOMPHALOS

This is a sporadic abnormality with a birth prevalence of about 1 in 4000. At 8–10 weeks of gestation, all fetuses demonstrate herniation of the midgut, visualized by ultrasound as a hyperechogenic mass in the base of the umbilical cord; retraction into the abdominal cavity occurs at 10–12 weeks and it is completed by 11 weeks and 5 days[31,70,71].

In the studies on chromosomally normal fetuses with increased nuchal translucency (Tables 1 and 2), the prevalence of exomphalos (11 in 4626), was higher than that expected in the general population[6,8,17,20,22]. Although one study reported that, in fetuses with exomphalos, increased nuchal translucency signifies an underlying chromosomal defect[31], it appears that, even in chromosomally normal fetuses with enlarged translucency, the prevalence of exomphalos is about 10 times higher than in the general population.

ACHONDROGENESIS TYPE II

This is a lethal, autosomal recessive skeletal dysplasia with a birth prevalence of about 1 in 40 000. In the second trimester, the characteristic sonographic features of achondrogenesis type II are severe shortening of the limbs, narrow thorax, hypomineralization of the vertebral bodies but normal mineralization of the skull, and hydrops. In achondrogenesis type I, which is more rare and is also autosomal recessive with severe shortening of the limbs, there is poor mineralization of both the skull and vertebral bodies as well as rib fractures.

In the studies reporting on chromosomally normal fetuses with increased nuchal translucency (Table 1), there was one case with the condition[9]. Additionally, there are two case reports on the first-trimester sonographic diagnosis of achondrogenesis type II in high-risk pregnancies; both fetuses had increased nuchal translucency and short limbs that were abnormally positioned, with lack of movement[32,33].

ACHONDROPLASIA

This autosomal dominant syndrome has a birth prevalence of about 1 in 26 000, but the majority of cases represent new mutations. The characteristic features include short limbs, lumbar lordosis, short hands and fingers, macrocephaly and depressed nasal bridge. Intelligence and life expectancy are normal. Prenatally, limb shortening usually becomes apparent only after 22 weeks of gestation.

In the studies reporting on chromosomally normal fetuses with increased nuchal translucency (Table 1), there were two cases with the condition[13,21].

ASPHYXIATING THORACIC DYSTROPHY

Asphyxiating thoracic dystrophy or Jeune's syndrome is an autosomal recessive condition with a birth prevalence of about 1 in 70 000. The characteristic features are narrow chest and rhizomelic limb shortening. There is a variable phenotypic expression and, consequently, the prognosis varies from neonatal death, due to pulmonary hypoplasia, to normal survival. Limb shortening is mild to moderate and this may not become apparent until after 24 weeks of gestation.

In a case report of Jeune's syndrome, routine ultrasound examination at 14 weeks demonstrated increased nuchal translucency (5.8 mm) and the femur length was on the 5th centile for gestation; repeat ultrasonography at 22 weeks showed a short narrow thorax and the length of all limbs was well below the 5th centile[34].

BECKWITH–WIEDEMANN SYNDROME

This is a usually sporadic and occasionally familial syndrome with a birth prevalence of about 1 in 14 000. It is characterized by macrosomia and hyperplasia and/or hypertrophy of the tongue, kidneys, adrenals, and pancreas, exomphalos and neonatal hypoglycemia and polycythemia. In some cases, there is mental handicap, which is thought to be secondary to inadequately treated hypoglycemia. About 5% of affected individuals develop tumors during childhood, most commonly nephroblastoma and hepatoblastoma.

In The Fetal Medicine Foundation Project (Table 2), one of the fetuses with increased nuchal translucency and exomphalos had Beckwith–Wiedemann syndrome[22].

BLOMSTRAND OSTEOCHONDRODYSPLASIA

This is a rare, lethal, autosomal recessive skeletal dysplasia characterized by severe shortening of all long bones, increased bone density, small oral cavity with protuberant tongue and hemosiderosis of the liver.

In a case report of a 12-week fetus with the syndrome, from a high-risk pregnancy, there was shortening of all limbs, narrow chest and increased nuchal translucency (6.3 mm); after termination of the pregnancy, pathological examination demonstrated thickening of periostal bone of the metaphyses and diaphyses and hemosiderosis of the liver[35].

BODY STALK ANOMALY

This lethal, sporadic abnormality, characterized by the presence of a major abdominal wall defect, severe kyphoscoliosis and a rudimentary umbilical cord, has a birth prevalence of about 1 in 15 000. The pathogenesis is uncertain but possible causes include abnormal folding of the trilaminar embryo during the first 4 weeks of development, early amnion rupture with amniotic band syndrome, and early generalized compromise of embryonic blood flow.

In the studies on chromosomally normal fetuses with increased nuchal translucency (Tables 1 and 2), the prevalence of body stalk anomaly (12 in 4626) was higher than that expected in the general population[11,13,22]. In a screening study involving ultrasound examinations at 11–14 weeks and 18–20 weeks of gestation in 3991 patients, there were two cases of body stalk anomaly and they were both diagnosed at the early scan; in one of the cases, there was increased nuchal translucency thickness[13].

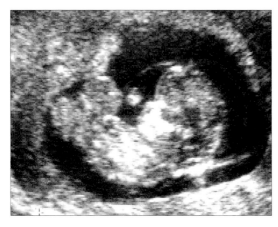

Figure 3 Body stalk anomaly in a 12-week fetus. The lower part of the body is in the celomic cavity and the upper part in the amniotic cavity

In a multicenter study for chromosomal defects by nuchal translucency thickness and maternal age, 106 727 fetuses were examined and 14 of these had body stalk anomaly[36]. The ultrasonographic features were a major abdominal wall defect, severe kyphoscoliosis and a short umbilical cord. In all cases, the upper half of the fetal body was in the amniotic cavity, whereas the lower part was in the celomic cavity, suggesting that early amnion rupture before obliteration of the celomic cavity is a possible cause of the syndrome. Although the nuchal translucency thickness was increased in 71% of the fetuses, the karyotype was normal in all cases[36].

CAMPOMELIC DYSPLASIA

This is a rare, lethal, autosomal recessive syndrome characterized by shortening and bowing of the lower limbs, growth deficiency of prenatal onset, large calvarium with disproportionately small face and narrow chest. Some of the affected genetically male individuals show a female phenotype. Patients usually die in the neonatal period from pulmonary hypoplasia.

In the studies reporting on chromosomally normal fetuses with increased nuchal translucency (Table 1), there was one case with the condition[6].

ECTRODACTYLY-ECTODERMAL DYSPLASIA-CLEFT PALATE (EEC) SYNDROME

This is a rare autosomal dominant condition with a wide variability in phenotypic expression. It is characterized by ectrodactyly (split hand and foot), facial cleft (lip and/or palate) and ectrodermal dysplasia (anomalies of hair, teeth, nails, nasolacrimal ducts and sweat glands).

In the studies reporting on chromosomally normal fetuses with increased nuchal translucency (Table 1), there was one case with the condition[14]. Additionally, there is one case report of EEC syndrome presenting with increased nuchal translucency, oligodactyly and umbilical cord cyst at 14 weeks; after termination of pregnancy, pathological examination demonstrated coarctation of the aorta[37]. There is another case report on the early diagnosis of the syndrome, but the study does not comment on nuchal translucency measurement; routine ultrasound examination at 14 weeks demonstrated lobster-claw deformities of the hands and feet and facial clefting[72] . Pathological examination after termination of the pregnancy confirmed the diagnosis. Subsequently, examination of the parents demonstrated no physical abnormalities, but the mother had microdontia of the lateral upper incisors which were crowned at the age of 15 years[72].

FETAL AKINESIA DEFORMATION SEQUENCE (FADS)

This is a heterogeneous group of conditions resulting in multiple joint contractures, including bilateral talipes and fixed flexion or extension deformities of the hips, knees, elbows and wrists. This sequence includes congenital lethal arthrogryposis, multiple pterygium and Pena–Shokeir syndromes. Pathological studies have reported that these features are frequently associated with fetal myopathy, neuropathy or an underlying connective tissue abnormality. Prenatal diagnosis is usually made by ultrasonography during the second or third trimesters of pregnancy and is based on the demonstration of the skeletal deformities; in about one-quarter of the cases, there is nuchal edema[38].

In the studies on chromosomally normal fetuses with increased nuchal translucency (Tables 1 and 2), the prevalence of FADS (nine in 4626) was higher than that expected in the general population[8,17,22]. A case report of a 12-week fetus in a woman with a previous pregnancy affected by FADS reported akinesia, extention of the hips and flexion of the knees; the study did not comment on the measurement of nuchal translucency[73].

Hyett et al.[38] examined at 11–13 weeks five pregnancies with a previous history of FADS. In three cases with no obvious fetal defects and normal nuchal translucency thickness, there were no abnormal findings at the subsequent scans and healthy infants were delivered at term. In two cases, the fetal nuchal translucency thickness was increased and detailed examination demonstrated bilateral fixed flexion deformities of the hands, wrists, elbows and knees, as well as severe talipes. In both cases, chorionic villus sampling was carried out and the fetal karyotype was normal. These findings, as

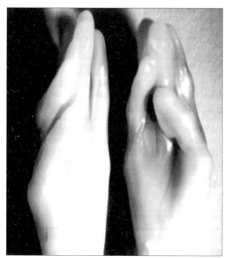

Figure 4 Photomicrograph of the hands of a fetus with fetal akinesia deformation sequence presenting at 13 weeks with increased nuchal translucency thickness

well as the known association between FADS and nuchal edema or hydrops in the second and third trimesters, suggest that, at least in some of the cases, there is increased nuchal translucency thickness at the 11–14-week scan.

FRYN SYNDROME

This is a usually lethal autosomal recessive disorder with a birth prevalence of about 1 in 15 000. It is characterized by the presence of diaphragmatic hernia, digital defects, coarse face and short webbed neck.

In two case reports on the first-trimester presentation of this syndrome, both fetuses had increased nuchal translucency[39,40]. In the first case, the fetus had a large nuchal translucency at 12 weeks, which partially resolved by 16 weeks[39]. At 20 weeks, diaphragmatic hernia, pleural effusions and ascites were detected and the limb measurements were on the 5th centile. At 24 weeks, polyhydramnios developed. The infant died in the neonatal period after delivery at 34 weeks, and pathological examination suggested the diagnosis of Fryn syndrome; there was a large diaphragmatic hernia, short neck with redundant nuchal skin, facial dysmorphism, hypertrichosis and distal digital hypoplasia[39]. In the second case, there was a family history of Fryn syndrome; at 12 weeks there was a large translucency and, after termination, pathological examination demonstrated facial cleft, pterygia of the upper limbs, syndactyly of the hands, oligodactyly of the feet, atresia of the aortic arch and truncus arteriosus with ventricular septal defect[40].

GM1-GANGLIOSIDOSIS

This is a rare, lethal, autosomal recessive condition resulting from β-galactosidase deficiency. It is characterized by visceromegaly, generalized edema and progressive neurological deterioration, resulting in early and severe retardation of both motor and mental development. Death occurs within the first 10 years of life from chest infections.

In the studies reporting on chromosomally normal fetuses with increased nuchal translucency (Table 1), there was one case with the condition[14].

HYDROLETHALUS SYNDROME

This is a rare, lethal, autosomal recessive condition characterized by hydrocephalus, absent corpus callosum, facial cleft, micrognathia, polydactyly, talipes and cardiac septal defects. The brain hemispheres lie separated from each other at the bottom of the skull and the lateral ventricles open medially into the fluid-filled space between and on the top of the hemispheres.

Ammala and Salonen[41] reported the ultrasound diagnosis at 12 weeks in a high-risk pregnancy from Finland, where the condition may be more common. There were abnormal brain structures with mid-line echoes only at the bottom of the skull and a large cyst in the upper posterior part of the brain and talipes; in addition, there was increased nuchal translucency[41]. In another non-Finnish family at high risk for this syndrome, ultrasound examination at 11 weeks demonstrated increased nuchal translucency, a keyhole defect of the skull in the occipital region and talipes[42].

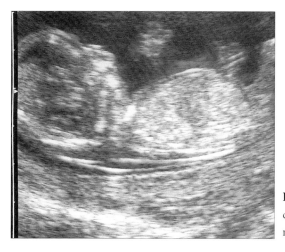

Figure 5 Increased nuchal translucency in a 13-week chromosomally normal fetus with severe micrognathia

JARCHO–LEVIN SYNDROME

This is a heterogeneous disorder that is characterized by vertebral and rib abnormalities. An autosomal recessive type (spondylothoracic dysplasia) is characterized by a constricted, short thorax and lethal respiratory insufficiency in infancy. Another type (spondylocostal dysplasia), in which most cases are autosomal recessive but a few are autosomal dominant, is associated with survival to adult life but with some degree of physical disability. In this type, there are other abnormalities, such as caudal agenesis and diaphragmatic hernia.

In The Fetal Medicine Foundation Project (Table 2), there were two cases of this syndrome; in one the diagnosis was made postnatally and in the other by pathological examination after termination of the pregnancy for severe scoliosis at 12 weeks[22]. In a report on the sonographic features of the syndrome in three affected fetuses at 12 weeks of gestation, there was misalignment of the cervical spine and ribs; additionally, one of the fetuses had increased nuchal translucency at 12 weeks but this resolved spontaneously by 15 weeks[43]. In another case report, a fetus with spondylocostal dysplasia presented at 12 weeks with increased nuchal translucency and a large cyst occupying the left abdominal and thoracic cavity; at 14 weeks, it was additionally noted that the fetus had thoracic scoliosis and misalignment of the cervical spine and ribs[44]. The pregnancy was terminated and pathological examination confirmed the prenatal findings; the abdominal cyst was a grossly distended stomach that had partly herniated into the chest through a large left-sided diaphragmatic hernia.

JOUBERT SYNDROME

This is a rare, lethal, autosomal recessive condition characterized by partial or complete absence of the cerebellar vermis. It is associated with profound mental retardation and developmental delay. Death usually occurs in the first 5 years of life.

In the studies on chromosomally normal fetuses with increased nuchal translucency (Tables 1 and 2), the prevalence of Joubert syndrome (two in 4626) was higher than that expected in the general population[12,22].

MECKEL–GRUBER SYNDROME

This lethal, autosomal recessive condition, with a birth prevalence of about 1 in 10 000, is characterized by the triad of encephalocele, bilateral polycystic kidneys and polydactyly.

In one case report of a fetus with Meckel–Gruber syndrome, there was increased nuchal translucency[45], but in another study, reporting on five affected fetuses, none had increased translucency[46].

NANCE–SWEENEY SYNDROME

This is a very rare, autosomal recessive syndrome characterized by short limbs, vertebral abnormalities, deafness and flat face with depressed nasal bridge. Intelligence and life expectancy are normal.

In The Fetal Medicine Foundation Project (Table 2), there was one case of Nance–Sweeney syndrome presenting with increased nuchal translucency (5 mm) at 11 weeks, which resolved by 20 weeks; the diagnosis of the syndrome was made postnatally[24].

NOONAN SYNDROME

This is an autosomal dominant condition with wide variability in expression but about 50% of cases represent new mutations. The birth prevalence is about 1 in 2000. It is characterized by lymphedema, thought to be due to dysplasia of the lymphatic system, short and webbed neck, short stature, heart defects, most commonly pulmonary valve stenosis, shield chest, hypertelorism and low set ears. Life expectancy is probably normal in those individuals without severe heart disease. Mild mental retardation is present in about one-third of cases.

In The Fetal Medicine Foundation Project (Table 2), there was only one case of Noonan syndrome, but, in the other studies on a total of 510 chromosomally normal fetuses with increased nuchal translucency, there were five cases of the syndrome (Table 1)[3,7,12,14,19,22].

OSTEOGENESIS IMPERFECTA TYPE II

This is a lethal skeletal dysplasia with a birth prevalence of about 1 in 60 000. The majority of cases are new mutations of the genes encoding for polypeptide chains 1 and 2 of collagen type I. Recurrence (6–7%) is usually due to parental mosaicism (somatic or germ-line), although, in a small number of families, autosomal recessive inheritance has been observed[74]. In the second trimester, the characteristic sonographic features are short limbs and ribs with multiple fractures and hypomineralization of the skull. Death occurs either prenatally or shortly after birth because of respiratory failure. In high-risk pregnancies, prenatal diagnosis can be made by chorionic villus sampling and DNA analysis or demonstration of abnormal collagen production by cultured fibroblasts.

Makrydimas et al.[48] reported two cases of ostegenesis imperfecta type II in low-risk patients presenting with increased nuchal translucency (3.4 mm and 4.4 mm, repectively) at 11 weeks. In the first case, repeat ultrasound examination at 15 weeks showed multiple fractures, shortening of long bones, rib fractures and hypomineralization of the skull. The diagnosis of osteogenesis imperfecta type II was made and this was confirmed radiographically and by pathological examination after termination of the pregnancy. In the second case, there was obvious shortening of all long bones and ribs at the 11-week scan. There are another three reported cases of osteogenesis imperfecta type II diagnosed in the first trimester, by demonstration of short, fractured femurs and hypomineralization of the skull, but in these reports there is no comment on the measurement of nuchal translucency[75–77].

PERLMAN SYNDROME

This is a rare, autosomal recessive condition characterized by macrosomia, nephro-megaly and depressed nasal bridge. The condition is similar to Beckwith–Wiedemann syndrome but they differ in their facial features. Fetal and neonatal mortality is more than 60% and, in survivors, there is a high incidence of neurodevelopmental delay.

In a case report of Perlman syndrome, the fetus presented with increased nuchal translucency (5 mm) at 11 weeks, which resolved by 23 weeks[49]. Serial scans demon-strated progressive macrosomia and enlarged kidneys; delivery was carried out at 32 weeks for macrosomia (birth weight 2.8 kg) and the baby died in the neonatal period.

ROBERTS SYNDROME

This is a rare, autosomal recessive condition characterized by symmetrical limb defects of variable severity (tetraphocomelia), facial cleft, hypertelorism, microcephaly and growth retardation. The condition is associated with the cytogenetic finding of pre-mature centromere separation and puffing.

In a case report of an 11-week affected fetus from a high-risk pregnancy, there was tetraphocomelia and increased nuchal translucency[50]. Another study on the diagnosis of Roberts syndrome reported short limbs in two fetuses at 10 weeks and tetraphocomelia in a third case at 13 weeks; this study did not examine the possible association with increased nuchal translucency[78].

SHORT-RIB POLYDACTYLY SYNDROME

This is a rare, autosomal recessive, lethal skeletal dysplasia, characterized by short limbs, narrow thorax and post-axial polydactyly. Associated anomalies are frequently found, including congenital heart disease, polycystic kidneys and intestinal atresia. Four different types have been recognized. Type I (Saldino–Noonan) has narrow metaphyses; type II (Majewski) has cleft lip and palate and disproportionally shortened tibiae; type III (Naumoff) has wide metaphyses with spurs; type IV (Beemer–Langer) is characterized by median cleft lip, small chest with extremely short ribs, pro-tuberant abdomen with umbilical hernia and ambiguous genitalia in some 46,XY individuals.

In a case report of a 13-week fetus with short-rib polydactyly syndrome type I, from a high-risk pregnancy, a narrow chest, short limbs, polydactyly and increased nuchal translucency were present[51].

SMITH–LEMLI–OPITZ SYNDROME

This is an autosomal recessive condition with a birth prevalence of about 1 in 20 000. It is associated with a high perinatal and infant mortality. The features include severe mental retardation, characteristic minor facial anomalies, cleft palate, polydactyly and syndactyly, cardiac defects and, in the male, ambiguous or female external genitalia, and deficiency of the enzyme 7-dehydrocholesterol reductase.

In The Fetal Medicine Foundation Project (Table 2), there were three cases of Smith–Lemli–Opitz syndrome[22]. In one case, the diagnosis was made postnatally, and, in the second, a chromosomally normal male fetus was found by ultrasonography at 20 weeks to have female external genitalia; examination of cultured skin fibroblasts demonstrated increased levels of 7-dehydrocholesterol[53]. In the third case, the mother had a previous pregnancy resulting in unexplained neonatal death and the diagnosis of Smith–Lemli–Opitz syndrome in the index pregnancy was made by DNA analysis after chorionic villus sampling for increased (6 mm) nuchal translucency. There are also two case reports on the first-trimester sonographic diagnosis of the condition in high-risk pregnancies and in both cases there was increased nuchal translucency[52,54].

SPINAL MUSCULAR ATROPHY TYPE 1 (WERDNIG–HOFFMANN DISEASE)

This is a lethal, autosomal recessive condition with a birth prevalence of about 1 in 25 000. It is characterized by degeneration of anterior horn cells of the spinal cord and brain stem with subsequent muscular hypotonia and atrophy. The onset of symptoms may be intrauterine with a decrease in fetal movements. Death, which occurs in the first 2 years of life, is usually due to respiratory failure.

There are five reported cases of spinal muscular atrophy type 1 presenting in the first trimester with increased nuchal translucency. In two cases, the diagnosis was made antenatally by chorionic villus sampling in patients with a family history of the condition and the pregnancies were terminated[14,55]. In the other three cases, the babies died in the neonatal period[16,22,56].

THANATOPHORIC DYSPLASIA

This is a sporadic condition with a birth prevalence of about 1 in 10 000. The term derives from the Greek, meaning death-bearing. It is characterized by severe shortening of the limbs which are bowed, narrow thorax with short ribs and enlarged head with prominent forehead; in some cases, there is a cloverleaf skull. The condition is lethal, usually in the neonatal period.

In The Fetal Medicine Foundation Project (Table 2), there was one case of thanatophoric dysplasia presenting with increased nuchal translucency (3 mm) at 11 weeks; severe limb shortening and narrow thorax were detected at 17 weeks[22]. There is a case report on the first-trimester diagnosis of the condition, by the detection of a narrow chest with short and bowed femurs; there is no comment on nuchal translucency measurement[79].

TRIGONOCEPHALY 'C' SYNDROME

This is an extremely rare, autosomal recessive condition characterized by trigonocephaly, short nose, prominent maxilla, joint deformities and loose skin due to hyperelasticity. About half of the affected individuals die in infancy while survivors are severely mentally handicapped with progressive microcephaly.

In The Fetal Medicine Foundation Project (Table 2), there was one case of trigonocephaly 'C' syndrome presenting at 13 weeks with increased nuchal translucency (3.3 mm); the diagnosis of the condition was made postnatally[22].

VACTERL ASSOCIATION

The acronym VACTERL is used to describe a rare, sporadic association of defects including vertebral abnormalities, anal atresia, cardiac defects, tracheo-esophageal fistula with esophageal atresia, radial and renal defects. The prognosis of each patient depends on the particular combination and severity of the abnormalities present. Mental function is usually normal.

In The Fetal Medicine Foundation Project (Table 2), there were two cases of the syndrome presenting at 12 weeks with increased nuchal translucency (2.8 mm and 3.0 mm, respectively); the diagnosis of VACTERL association was made prenatally in one case and postnatally in the other case[22].

ZELLWEGER SYNDROME

This lethal, autosomal recessive syndrome has a birth prevalence of about 1 in 25 000. It is characterized by absence or marked decrease in peroxisomes, resulting in profound muscular hypotonia. Other features include dolichoturricephaly, hypertelorism, cataracts, brain abnormalities, cardiac defects, hepatomegaly, and growth retardation.

Death occurs in the first 2 years of life, most commonly due to chest infections and liver failure.

In a case report of Zellweger syndrome, the fetus had increased nuchal translucency (6 mm) at 12 weeks and pericardial effusion at 20 weeks; the diagnosis of the condition was made postnatally[57].

REFERENCES

1. Nicolaides KH, Azar G, Byrne D, Mansur C, Marks K. Fetal nuchal translucency: ultrasound screening for chromosomal defects in first trimester of pregnancy. *Br Med J* 1992;304:867–9

2. Snijders RJM, Noble P, Sebire N, Souka A, Nicolaides KH. UK multicentre project on assessment of risk of trisomy 21 by maternal age and fetal nuchal translucency thickness at 10–14 weeks of gestation. *Lancet* 1998;352:343–6

3. Johnson MP, Johnson A, Holzgreve W, Isada NB, Wapner RJ, Treadwell MC, Heeger S, Evans M. First-trimester simple hygroma: cause and outcome. *Am J Obstet Gynecol* 1993;168:156–61

4. Trauffer ML, Anderson CE, Johnson A, Heeger S, Morgan P, Wapner RJ. The natural history of euploid pregnancies with first-trimester cystic hygromas. *Am J Obstet Gynecol* 1994;170:1279–84

5. Shulman LP, Emerson DS, Grevengood C, Felker RE, Gross SJ, Phillips OP, Elias S. Clinical course and outcome of fetuses with isolated cystic nuchal lesions and normal karyotypes detected in the first trimester. *Am J Obstet Gynecol* 1994;171:1278–81

6. Hafner E, Schuchter K, Liebhart E, Philipp K. Results of routine fetal nuchal translucency measurement at weeks 10–13 in 4,233 unselected pregnant women. *Prenat Diagn* 1998;18:29–34

7. van Zalen-Sprock RM, van Vugt JMG, van Geijn HP. First-trimester diagnosis of cystic hygroma – course and outcome. *Am J Obstet Gynecol* 1992;167:94–8

8. Ville Y, Lalondrelle C, Doumerc S, Daffos F, Frydman R, Oury JF, Dumez Y. First-trimester diagnosis of nuchal anomalies: significance and fetal outcome. *Ultrasound Obstet Gynecol* 1992;2:314–16

9. Hewitt B. Nuchal translucency in the first trimester. *Aust NZ J Obstet Gynaecol* 1993;33:389–91

10. Salvesen DR, Goble O. Early amniocentesis and fetal nuchal translucency in women requesting karyotyping for advanced maternal age. *Prenat Diagn* 1995;15:971–4

11. Hewitt BG, de Crespigny L, Sampson AJ, Ngu ACC, Shekleton P, Robinson HP. Correlation between nuchal thickness and abnormal karyotype in first trimester fetuses. *MJA* 1996;165:365–8

12. Reynders CS, Pauker SP, Benacerraf BR. First trimester isolated fetal nuchal lucency: significance and outcome. *J Ultrasound Med* 1997;16:101–5

13. Hernadi L, Torocsik M. Screening for fetal anomalies in the 12th week of pregnancy by transvaginal sonography in an unselected population. *Prenat Diagn* 1997;17:753–9

14. Bilardo CM, Pajkrt E, de Graaf IM, Mol BWJ, Bleker OP. Outcome of fetuses with enlarged nuchal translucency and normal karyotype. *Ultrasound Obstet Gynecol* 1998;11:401–6

15. Pajkrt E, van Lith JMM, Mol BWJ, Bleker OP, Bilardo CM. Screening for Down's syndrome by fetal nuchal translucency measurement in a general obstetric population. *Ultrasound Obstet Gynecol* 1998;12:163–9

16. van Vugt JMG, Tinnemans BWS, van Zalen-Sprock RM. Outcome and early childhood follow-up of chromosomally normal fetuses with increased nuchal translucency at 10–14 weeks' gestation. *Ultrasound Obstet Gynecol* 1998;11:407–9

17. Nadel A, Bromley B, Benacerraf BR. Nuchal thickening or cystic hygromas in first- and early second-trimester fetuses: prognosis and outcome. *Obstet Gynecol* 1993;82:43–8

18. Moselhi M, Thilaganathan B. Nuchal translucency: a marker for the antenatal diagnosis of aortic coarctation. *Br J Obstet Gynaecol* 1996;103:1044–5

19. Thilaganathan B, Slack A, Wathen NC. Effect of first-trimester nuchal translucency on second trimester maternal serum biochemical screening for Down's syndrome. *Ultrasound Obstet Gynecol* 1997;10:261–4

20. Adekunle O, Gopee A, El-Sayed M, Thilaganathan B. Increased first-trimester nuchal translucency: pregnancy and infant outcomes after routine screening for Down's syndrome in an unselected antenatal population. *Br J Radiol* 1999;72:457–60

21. Fukada Y, Yasumizu T, Takizawa M, Amemiya A, Hoshi K. The prognosis of fetuses with transient nuchal translucency in the first and early second trimester. *Acta Obstet Gynecol Scand* 1998;76: 913–16

22. Souka AP, Snidjers RJM, Novakov A, Soares W, Nicolaides KH. Defects and syndromes in chromosomally normal fetuses with increased nuchal translucency thickness at 10–14 weeks of gestation. *Ultrasound Obstet Gynecol* 1998;11:391–400

23. Pandya PP, Kondylios A, Hilbert L, Snijders RJM, Nicolaides KH. Chromosomal defects and outcome in 1015 fetuses with increased nuchal translucency. *Ultrasound Obstet Gynecol* 1995;5:15–19

24. Brady AF, Pandya PP, Yuksel B, Greenough A, Patton MA, Nicolaides KH. Outcome of chromosomally normal livebirths with increased fetal nuchal translucency at 10–14 weeks' gestation. *J Med Genet* 1998;35:222–4

25. Gembruch U, Knopfle G, Chatterjee M, Bald R, Hansmann M. First-trimester diagnosis of fetal congenital heart disease by transvaginal two-dimensional and Doppler echocardiography. *Obstet Gynecol* 1990;75:496–8

26. Gembruch U, Knopfle G, Bald R, Hansmann M. Early diagnosis of fetal congenital heart disease by transvaginal echocardiography. *Ultrasound Obstet Gynecol* 1993;3:310–17

27. Bronshtein M, Siegler E, Yoffe N, Zimmer EZ. Prenatal diagnosis of ventricular septal defect and overriding aorta at 14 weeks' gestation, using transvaginal sonography. *Prenat Diagn* 1990;10: 697–702

28. Achiron R, Rotstein Z, Lipitz S, Mashiach S, Hegesh J. First-trimester diagnosis of fetal congenital heart disease by transvaginal ultrasonography. *Obstet Gynecol* 1994;84:69–72

29. Sebire NJ, Snijders RJM, Davenport M, Greenough A, Nicolaides KH. Fetal nuchal translucency thickness at 10–14 weeks of gestation and congenital diaphragmatic hernia. *Obstet Gynecol* 1997; 90:943–7

30. Lam YH, Tang MHY, Yuen ST. Ultrasound diagnosis of fetal diaphragmatic hernia and complex congenital heart disease at 12 weeks' gestation – a case report. *Prenat Diagn* 1998;18:1159–62

31. van Zalen-Sprock RM, van Vugt JMG, van Geijn HP. First-trimester sonography of physiological midgut herniation and early diagnosis of omphalocele. *Prenat Diagn* 1997;17:511–18

32. Fisk NM, Vaughan J, Smidt M, Wigglesworth J. Transvaginal ultrasound recognition of nuchal oedema in the first-trimester diagnosis of achondrogenesis. *J Clin Ultrasound* 1991;19:586–90

33. Soothill PW, Vuthiwong C, Rees H. Achondrogenesis type 2 diagnosed by transvaginal ultrasound at 12 weeks of gestation. *Prenat Diagn* 1993;13:523–8

34. Ben Ami M, Perlitz Y, Haddad S, Matilsky M. Increased nuchal translucency is associated with asphyxiating thoracic dysplasia. *Ultrasound Obstet Gynecol* 1997;10:297–8

35. den Hollander NS, van der Harten HJ, Vermeij-Keers C, Niermeijer MF, Wladimiroff JW. First trimester diagnosis of Blomstrand lethal osteochondrodysplasia. *Am J Med Genet* 1997;73: 345–50

36. Daskalakis G, Sebire NJ, Jurkovic D, Snijders RJM, Nicolaides KH. Body stalk anomaly at 10–14 weeks of gestation. *Ultrasound Obstet Gynecol* 1997;10:416–18

37. Leung KY, MacLachlan NA, Sepulveda W. Prenatal diagnosis of ectrodactyly: the 'lobster claw' anomaly. *Ultrasound Obstet Gynecol* 1995;6:443–6

38. Hyett J, Noble P, Sebire NJ, Snijders RJM, Nicolaides KH. Lethal congenital arthrogryposis presents with increased nuchal translucency at 10–14 weeks of gestation. *Ultrasound Obstet Gynecol* 1997;9: 310–13

39. Bulas D, Saal H, Allen JF, Kapur S, Nies BM, Newman K. Cystic hygroma and congenital diaphragmatic hernia: early prenatal sonographic evaluation of Fryn's syndrome. *Prenat Diagn* 1992;12 :867–75

40. Hosli IM, Tercanli S, Rehder H, Holzgreve W. Cystic hygroma as an early first-trimester ultrasound marker for recurrent Fryns' syndrome. *Ultrasound Obstet Gynecol* 1997;10:422–4

41. Ammala P, Salonen R. First-trimester diagnosis of hydrolethalus syndrome. *Ultrasound Obstet Gynecol* 1995;5:60–2

42. de Ravelle TJL, van der Griendt MC, Evan P, Wright CA. Hydrolethalus syndrome in a non-Finnish family: confirmation of the entity and early prenatal diagnosis. *Prenat Diagn* 1999;19: 279–81

43. Eliyahu S, Weiner E, Lahav D, Shalev E. Early sonographic diagnosis of Jarcho-Levin syndrome: a prospective screening program in one family. *Ultrasound Obstet Gynecol* 1997;9:314–18

44. Lam YH, Eik-Nes SH, Tang MHY, Lee CP, Nicholls JM. Prenatal sonographic features of spondylocostal dysostosis and diaphragmatic hernia in the first trimester. *Ultrasound Obstet Gynecol* 1999;13:213–15

45. Quintero R, Abuhamad A, Hobbins JC, Mahoney MJ. Transabdominal thin-gauge embryofetoscopy: a technique for early prenatal diagnosis and its use in the diagnosis of a case of Meckel–Gruber syndrome. *Am J Obstet Gynecol* 1993;168:1552–7

46. Sepulveda W, Sebire NJ, Souka A, Snijders RJM, Nicolaides KH. Diagnosis of the Meckel–Gruber syndrome at eleven to fourteen weeks' gestation. *Am J Obstet Gynecol* 1997;176:316–19

47. Sebire NJ, von Kaisenberg C, Rubio C, Snijders RJM, Nicolaides KH. Fetal megacystis at 10–14 weeks of gestation. *Ultrasound Obstet Gynecol* 1996;8:387–90

48. Makrydimas G, Souka A, Skentou H, Lolis D, Nicolaides KH. Osteogenesis imperfecta and other skeletal dysplasias present with increased nuchal translucency in the first trimester: two case-reports and review of the literature. *Am J Med Genet* 1999:in press

49. van der Stege, van Eyck J, Arabin B. Prenatal ultrasound observation in subsequent pregnancies with Perlman syndrome. *Ultrasound Obstet Gynecol* 1998;11:149–51

50. Petrikovsky BM, Gross B, Bialer M, Solamanzadeh K, Simhaee E. Prenatal diagnosis of pseudothalidomide syndrome in consecutive pregnancies of a consanguineous couple. *Ultrasound Obstet Gynecol* 1997;10:425–8

51. Hill LM, Leary J. Transvaginal sonographic diagnosis of short-rib polydactyly dysplasia at 13 weeks' gestation. *Prenat Diagn* 1998;18:1198–201

52. Hobbins JC, Jones OW, Gottesfeld S, Persutte W. Transvaginal sonography and transabdominal embryoscopy in the first-trimester diagnosis of Smith–Lemli–Opitz syndrome, type 2. *Am J Obstet Gynecol* 1994;171:546–9

53. Hyett JA, Clayton PT, Moscoso G, Nicolaides KH. Increased first trimester nuchal translucency as a prenatal manifestation of Smith–Lemli–Opitz syndrome. *Am J Med Genet* 1995;58:374–6

54. Sharp P, Haant E, Fletcher JM, Khong TY, Carey WF. First-trimester diagnosis of Smith–Lemli–Opitz syndrome. *Prenat Diagn* 1997;17:355–61

55. Rijhsinghani A, Yankowitz J, Howser D, Williamson R. Sonographic and maternal serum screening abnormalities in fetuses affected by spinal muscular atrophy. *Prenat Diagn* 1997;17: 166–9

56. Stiller RJ, Lieberson D, Herzlinger R, Siddiqui D, Laifer SA, Whetham JCG. The association of increased fetal nuchal translucency and spinal muscular atrophy type I. *Prenat Diagn* 1999;19: 587–9

57. de Graaf IM, Pajkrt E, Keessen M, Leschot NJ, Bilardo CM. Enlarged nuchal translucency and low serum protein concentration as possible markers for Zellweger syndrome. *Ultrasound Obstet Gynecol* 1999;13:268–70

58. Hyett JA, Moscoso G, Nicolaides KH. First trimester nuchal translucency and cardiac septal defects in fetuses with trisomy 21. *Am J Obstet Gynecol* 1995;172:1411–13

59. Hyett JA, Moscoso G, Nicolaides KH. Cardiac defects in first trimester fetuses with trisomy 18. *Fetal Diagn Ther* 1995;10:381–6

60. Hyett JA, Moscoso G, Nicolaides KH. Morphometric analysis of the great vessels in early fetal life. *Hum Reprod* 1995;10:3045–8

61. Hyett JA, Moscoso G, Nicolaides KH. Increased nuchal translucency in trisomy 21 fetuses: relation to narrowing of the aortic isthmus. *Hum Reprod* 1995;10:3049–51

62. Hyett JA, Moscoso G, Nicolaides KH. Abnormalities of the heart and great arteries in first trimester chromosomally abnormal fetuses. *Am J Med Genet* 1997;69:207–16

63. Hyett JA, Perdu M, Sharland GK, Snijders RJM, Nicolaides KH. Increased nuchal translucency at 10–14 weeks of gestation as a marker for major cardiac defects. *Ultrasound Obstet Gynecol* 1997;10: 242–6

64. Hyett JA, Perdu M, Sharland GK, Snijders RJM, Nicolaides KH. Using fetal nuchal translucency to screen for major congenital cardiac defects at 10–14 weeks of gestation: population based cohort study. *Br Med J* 1999:318:81–5

65. Zosmer N, Souter VL, Chan CSY, Huggon IC, Nicolaides KH. Early diagnosis of major cardiac defects in chromosomally normal fetuses with increased nuchal translucency. *Br J Obstet Gynaecol* 1999;106:829–33

66. Dolkart LA, Reimers FT. Transvaginal fetal echocardiography in early pregnancy: normative data. *Am J Obstet Gynecol* 1991;165:688–91

67. Carvahlo JS, Moscoso G, Ville Y. First trimester transabdominal fetal echocardiography. *Lancet* 1998;351:1023–7

68. Sharland G. First trimester transabdominal fetal echocardiography. *Lancet* 1998;351:1662

69. Thorpe-Beeston JG, Gosden CM, Nicolaides KH. Prenatal diagnosis of congenital diaphragmatic hernia: associated malformations and chromosomal defects. *Fetal Ther* 1989;4:21–8

70. Blaas HG, Eik-Nes SH, Kiserud T, Hellevik LR. Early development of the abdominal wall, stomach and heart from 7 to 12 weeks of gestation: a longitudinal ultrasound study. *Ultrasound Obstet Gynecol* 1995;6:240–9

71. Timor-Tritsch IE, Warren W, Peisner DB, Pirrone E. First-trimester midgut herniation: a high frequency transvaginal sonographic study. *Am J Obstet Gynecol* 1989;161:831–3

72. Bronshtein M, Gershoni-Baruch R. Prenatal transvaginal diagnosis of the ectrodactyly, ectodermal dysplasia, cleft palate (EEC) syndrome. *Prenat Diagn* 1993;13:519–22

73. Ajayi RA, Keen CE, Knott PD. Ultrasound diagnosis of the Rena Shokeir phenotype at 14 weeks of pregnancy. *Prenat Diagn* 1995;15:762–4

74. Byers PH, Tsipouras P, Bonadio JF, Starman BJ, Schwartz RC. Perinatal lethal osteogenesis imperfecta (OI type II): a biochemically heterogeneous disorder usually due to new mutations in the genes for type I collagen. *Am J Hum Gen* 1988;42:237–48

75. Stephens J D, Filly RA, Callen PW, Golbus MS. Prenatal diagnosis of osteogenesis imperfecta type 2 by real-time ultrasound. *Hum Genet* 1983;64:191–3

76. Bronshtein M, Weiner Z. Anencephaly in a fetus with osteogenesis imperfecta: early sonographic diagnosis by transvaginal sonography. *Prenat Diagn* 1992;12:831–4

77. Dimaio MS, Barth R, Koprivnikar KE, Sussman BL, Copel JA, Mahoney MJ, Byers PH, Cohn DH. First trimester prenatal diagnosis of osteogenesis imperfecta type 2 by DNA analysis and sonography. *Prenat Diagn* 1993;13:589–96

78. Otano L, Matayoshi T, Lippold S, Serafin E, Scarpati R, Gadow EC. Roberts syndrome: first trimester prenatal diagnosis by cytogenetics and ultrasound in affected and non-affected pregnancies. *Am J Hum Gen* 1993;53:1445

79. Benacerraf B, Lister J, Du Ponte BL. First-trimester diagnosis of fetal abnormalities. *J Reprod Med* 1988;9:777–80

3

Pathophysiology of increased nuchal translucency

The heterogeneity of conditions associated with increased nuchal translucency suggests that there may not be a single underlying mechanism for the collection of fluid in the skin of the fetal neck. Possible mechanisms include:

(1) Cardiac failure in association with abnormalities of the heart and great arteries;

(2) Venous congestion in the head and neck, due to constriction of the fetal body in amnion rupture sequence or superior mediastinal compression found in diaphragmatic hernia or the narrow chest in skeletal dysplasia;

(3) Altered composition of the extracellular matrix;

(4) Abnormal or delayed development of the lymphatic system;

(5) Failure of lymphatic drainage due to impaired fetal movements in various neuromuscular disorders;

(6) Fetal anemia or hypoproteinemia;

(7) Congenital infection, acting through anemia or cardiac dysfunction.

CARDIAC DYSFUNCTION

Pathological studies

Pathological studies of the heart and great arteries, after surgical termination of pregnancy in 112 chromosomally abnormal fetuses identified by nuchal translucency screening at 10–14 weeks of gestation, demonstrated abnormalities of the heart and great arteries in the majority of cases (Figures 1–9)[1]. The commonest cardiac lesion seen in trisomy 21 fetuses was an atrioventricular or ventricular septal defect. Trisomy 18 was associated with ventricular septal defects and/or polyvalvular abnormalities. In trisomy 13, there were atrioventricular or ventricular septal defects, valvular abnormalities and either narrowing of the isthmus or truncus arteriosus. Turner syndrome was associated with severe narrowing of the whole aortic arch.

In all four groups of chromosomally abnormal fetuses, the aortic isthmus was significantly narrower than in normal fetuses, and the degree of narrowing was significantly greater in fetuses with increased nuchal translucency thickness[1]. In trisomies 21 and 18, narrowing of the isthmus was associated with widening of the ascending aorta. Since blood flow is related to vessel diameter, widening of the ascending aorta and narrowing of the isthmus could result in overperfusion of the tissues of the head and neck, leading to edema. With advancing gestation, the diameter of the aortic isthmus increases more rapidly than the diameters of the aortic valve and distal ductus and, therefore, the hemodynamic consequences of narrowing of the isthmus may be overcome[2,3]. Since vascular resistance depends on vessel radius by a factor of 10^{-4} (equation of Hagen–Poisseuille), a small increase in the diameter of the aortic isthmus would result in a major reduction in vascular resistance and possible resolution of nuchal translucency. This hypothesis could offer an explanation for the gestational age-related spontaneous resolution of nuchal translucency; for example, abnormal nuchal fluid is observed in about 70% of trisomy 21 fetuses at 11 weeks of gestation but in only 30% of cases at the 20th week[4].

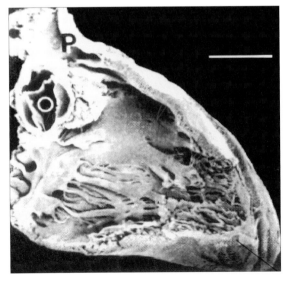

Figure 1 Scanning electron micrograph ($\times$ 25) showing the septal aspect of the right ventricle of a normal heart at 12 weeks of gestation. O, aorta; P, pulmonary trunk. Scale bar: 750 μm

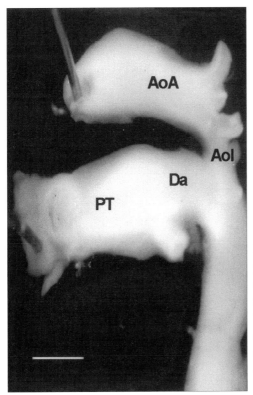

Figure 2 The ascending aorta (AoA), pulmonary trunk (PT), aortic isthmus (AoI) and ductus arteriosus (Da) from a trisomy 21-affected fetus at 14 weeks of gestation. The ascending aorta and the isthmus of the aorta show some developmental delay. The aortic isthmus is narrow compared to the distal ductus arteriosus, which is mildly dilated. Scale bar: 1 mm

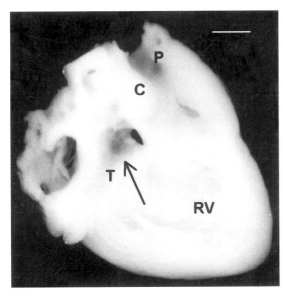

Figure 3 Photomicrograph showing a perimembranous ventricular septal defect (arrow), partially guarded by the septal leaflet of the tricuspid valve (T) of a 13-week trisomy 21 fetus. C, crista supraventricularis; P, pulmonary valve; RV, right ventricle. Scale bar: 1 mm

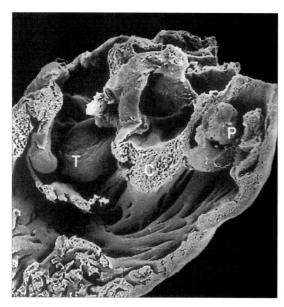

Figure 4 A scanning electron micrograph of the parietal aspect of the right ventricle showing marked dysplasia of both the pulmonary (P) and tricuspid (T) valves in the heart of a trisomy 18 fetus at 12 weeks of gestation. C, crista supraventricularis

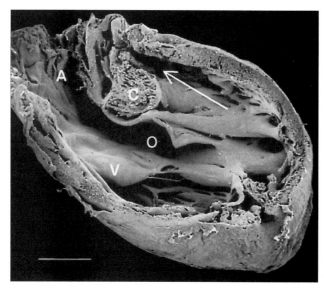

Figure 5 The septal aspects of the right ventricle showing a type 1 atrioventricular septal defect (O). The right ventricular outflow tract has collapsed partially during processing of the specimen (arrow). A, right atrium; V, common atrioventricular valve; C, crista supraventricularis. Scale bar: 500 μm

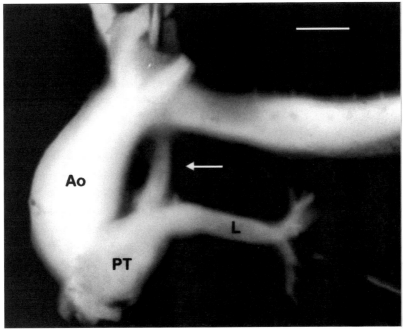

Figure 6   A hypoplastic pulmonary trunk (PT) and ductus arteriosus (arrow) in a trisomy 18 fetus at 13 weeks of gestation. The left pulmonary artery (L) and ascending aorta (Ao) are dilated. Scale bar: 1 mm

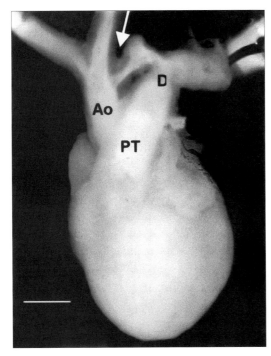

Figure 7   Tubular hypoplasia of the aortic isthmus (arrow) in this 12-week fetus with Turner syndrome. The ductus arteriosus (D) is dilated. PT, pulmonary trunk. Scale bar: 1 mm

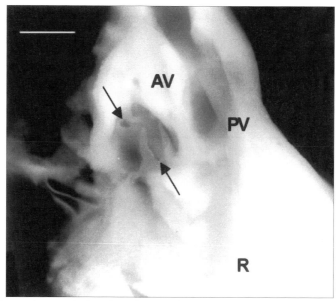

Figure 8 Photomicrograph showing a bicuspid aortic valve (AV) in a fetal heart at 11 weeks of gestation. Note the two commisures (arrows) at 10 and 4 o'clock. PV, pulmonary valve; R, right ventricle. Scale bar: 1 mm

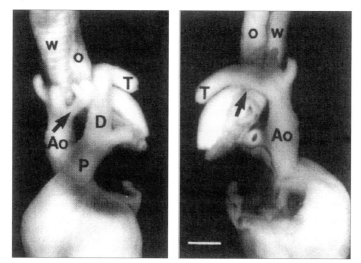

Figure 9 Photomicrograph of the heart and great vessels in a 12-week fetus, demonstrating a double aortic arch. On the left side, the aortic isthmus (arrow) is hypoplastic, whereas, on the right, the persisting right aortic arch (arrow) is dilated. Ao, ascending aorta; T, thoracic aorta; P, pulmonary trunk; D, ductus arteriosus; o, esophagus; w, trachea. Scale bar: 1 mm

In trisomy 13 and Turner syndrome, narrowing of the isthmus was accompanied by narrowing of the ascending aorta and, therefore development of increased nuchal translucency cannot be explained by overperfusion of the head and neck[1]. In the case of Turner syndrome, increased nuchal translucency is thought to represent overdistention of the jugular lymphatic sacs, as a consequence of failure of communication with the internal jugular vein[1]. It has been suggested that the associated cardiovascular malformations, primarily coarctation of the aorta and other defects in the spectrum of left heart obstruction, are the consequence of altered intracardiac blood flow, due to compression of the ascending aorta by the distended intrathoracic lymphatic channels[5].

The findings in the human of an association between increased nuchal translucency thickness and abnormalities of the heart and great arteries are consistent with animal studies. The trisomy 16 mouse (Figure 10), which is considered to be a good animal model for human trisomy 21, has a combination of abnormalities of lymph vessels, cardiovascular malformations and hypoplastic thymus, which have been attributed to impaired migration of neural crest cells[6]. These cells migrate from the embryonic neural tube and play a central role in the development of the cardiovascular system[7]. There is increasing evidence that many neural crest-related cardiovascular defects may

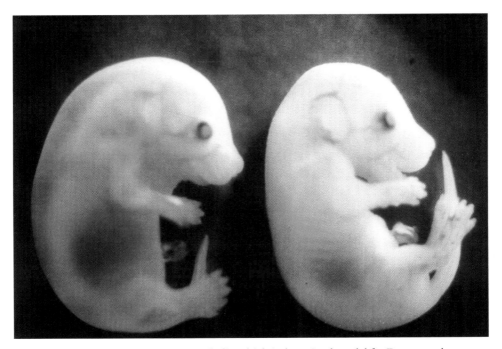

Figure 10 In the trisomy 16 mouse (left), which is the animal model for Down syndrome, on days 14, 15 and 16 of intrauterine life, there is a subcutaneous collection of fluid. On the right is the normal mouse. (Image kindly provided by Professor Buselmeier, University of Heidelberg)

be genetically based[8]. The genetic mechanism, whereby a series of different chromosomal defects interfere with neural crest cells to result in abnormalities of the aortic arch and cardiac defects, remains to be determined.

Doppler studies of the ductus venosus

The sphincter-like ductus venosus is an important regulator of the fetal circulation; it directs well-oxygenated umbilical venous blood to the coronary and cerebral circulation, by preferential streaming through the foramen ovale into the left atrium. Blood flow in the ductus is characterized by its high velocity during ventricular systole (S-wave) and diastole (D-wave) and by the presence of forward flow during atrial contraction (A-wave). In cardiac failure, with or without cardiac defects, there is absent or reversed A-wave[9]. A study, examining ductal flow at 11–14 weeks in fetuses with increased nuchal translucency, reported absent or reverse flow during atrial contraction in 57 of 63 (90.5%) chromosomally abnormal fetuses and in only 13 of 423 (3.1%) chromosomally normal fetuses (Figure 11)[10]. These findings suggest that a high proportion of chromosomally abnormal fetuses at 11–14 weeks of gestation demonstrate evidence of heart failure.

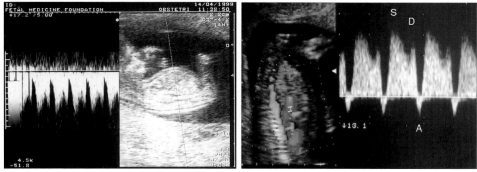

Figure 11 Ductal flow at 12 weeks of gestation. On the left is the flow velocity waveform of a normal fetus and on the right there is a reversed A-wave in a chromosomally abnormal fetus

Evidence that the heart failure is temporary is provided from those cases where chromosomal abnormalities were diagnosed in the first trimester but the parents chose to continue with the pregnancy. Thus, in a case of trisomy 21 with increased nuchal translucency at 13 weeks but no cardiac defect, there was abnormal ductal flow; at 15 weeks, both the translucency and the abnormal A-wave resolved[10]. Similarly, in a case of trisomy 18 with a membranous septal defect presenting at 13 weeks with increased nuchal translucency and reversed A-wave in the ductus, there was resolution of both the translucency and the abnormal ductal flow with advancing gestation[11].

Molecular biology studies

Atrial natriuretic peptide and brain natriuretic peptide (which are encoded on chromosome 1) are involved in fluid–electrolyte homeostasis, with potent diuretic–natriuretic and vasorelaxant effects. A number of extracardiac tissues have been shown to express atrial natriuretic peptide but synthesis and secretion are almost exclusively confined to the cardiac atria. The major source of circulating brain natriuretic peptide is the cardiac ventricles. A study of trisomic fetuses with increased nuchal translucency thickness reported increased levels of atrial and brain natriuretic peptide mRNA in fetal hearts[12]. On the basis of these results, it could be postulated that trisomic fetuses demonstrate heart strain. Certainly, in postnatal life, upregulation of natriuretic peptides is considered to occur as a compensatory mechanism to the characteristic changes of sodium retention and increased vascular resistance associated with congestive cardiac failure[13].

VENOUS CONGESTION IN THE HEAD AND NECK

Diaphragmatic hernia

Increased nuchal translucency thickness is present in about 40% of fetuses with diaphragmatic hernia, including more than 80% of those that result in neonatal death due to pulmonary hypoplasia and in about 20% of the survivors[14]. It is possible that, in those cases with increased nuchal translucency at 11–14 weeks, there is indeed intrathoracic herniation of the abdominal viscera during this stage of gestation, and the increased nuchal translucency may be the consequence of venous congestion in the head and neck due to mediastinal compression and impedence to venous return. In such cases, prolonged intrathoracic compression of the lungs causes pulmonary hypoplasia. In the cases where diaphragmatic hernia is associated with a good prognosis, the intrathoracic herniation of viscera may be delayed until the second or third trimesters of pregnancy[15]. An alternative hypothesis is that, in all cases of diaphragmatic hernia, there is intrathoracic herniation by 11 weeks, but increased nuchal translucency is only observed in those with sufficiently severe compression of the lungs to cause pulmonary hypoplasia. Screening for diaphragmatic hernia at the 11–14-week scan will help to determine which of the hypotheses is likely to be true.

Skeletal dysplasias

Intrathoracic compression may also be the underlying mechanism for the increased nuchal translucency observed in a wide range of skeletal dysplasias, which are associated with a narrow thoracic cage (see Chapter 2). However, in at least some of the cases, such as osteogenesis imperfecta, an additional or alternative mechanism for the increased translucency may be the altered composition of the extracellular matrix.

ALTERATION IN THE EXTRACELLULAR MATRIX

The extracellular matrix consists of ground substance (mucoproteins and mucopoly-saccharides) and collagen fibers. Collagens, which are produced by fibroblasts, are triple-helical proteins. Cells are fixed to the matrix and to each other by a group of molecules known as integrins (laminin and fibronectin).

Many of the component proteins of the extracellular matrix are encoded on chromosomes 21, 18 or 13 (Table 1). Immunohistochemical studies, using antibodies against collagen types I, III, IV, V and VI and against laminin and fibronectin to examine the skin of chromosomally abnormal fetuses, have demonstrated specific alterations of the extracellular matrix which may be attributed to gene dosage effects[16,17]. Thus, the dermis of trisomy 21 fetuses is rich in collagen type VI (Figure 12), whereas dermal fibroblasts of trisomy 13 fetuses demonstrate an abundance of collagen type IV and those of trisomy 18 fetuses an abundance of laminin[16].

Overexpression of several other genes found in chromosome 21 is thought to be the underlying mechanism for the phenotypic characteristics of trisomy 21. For example, overexpression of the amyloid precursor protein gene results in deposition of amyloid in the brain and early onset of Alzheimer's disease[18]. Additionally, transgenic mice that carry the *Ets2* gene, a proto-oncogene and transcription factor that is overexpressed in human trisomy 21, develop cranial and cervical skeletal abnormalities that are similar to those in Down's syndrome[19].

The molecule of collagen type VI, which forms microfibrils in tissues, is composed of three polypeptide chains $\alpha 1$, $\alpha 2$ and $\alpha 3$. In nuchal skin of trisomy 21 fetuses, the ratio of the expression of *COL6A1* (which is located on chromosome 21) to *COL6A3* (which is located on chromosome 2) is twice as high as in normal fetuses[16]. It is therefore possible that the composition and consequently the properties of collagen type VI are altered in trisomy 21 fetuses, leading to the accumulation of subcutaneous edema. Thus, collagen type VI binds to hyaluronic acid (a very large molecular weight polysaccharide)[20], which can entrap large amounts of solvent in the extracellular matrix. In postnatal life, conditions with increased levels of hyaluronic acid, such as inflammatory rheumatic diseases or cirrhotic liver disease, are associated with interstitial edema[21,22].

Table 1 Structural proteins of the extracellular matrix and gene loci. Genes that are likely to be overexpressed as a result of trisomies are indicated in bold type[17]

Component	Gene	Chromosome
Collagen type I	COL1A1	17q
Collagen type III	COL3A1	2q
Collagen type IV	**COL4A1**	**13q**
	COL4A2	**13q**
	COL4A3	2q
	COL4A4	2q
	COL4A5	Xq
	COL4A6	X
Collagen type V	COL5A1	9q
	COL5A2	22
Collagen type VI	**COL6A1**	**21q**
	COL6A2	**21q**
	COL6A3	2q
Laminin	**LAMA1**	**18p**
	LAMA2	6q
	LAMA3	**18q**
	LAMA4	6q
	LAMB1	7q
	LAMB2	1q
	LAMB2	3p
	LAMM	6q
Fibronectin	VNR (alpha)	2
	FNR (alpha)	12q

Immunohistochemical studies of fetal nuchal skin have demonstrated that, in fetuses with trisomy 21, there is a substantial increase in hyaluronic acid, whereas, in trisomies 18 and 13 and Turner syndrome, the amount is similar to that in chromosomally normal controls. The increased hyaluronic acid in trisomy 21 fetuses may be the consequence of increased synthesis or decreased degradation, but the gene loci for the enzymes involved in these processes have not yet been mapped. However, superoxide dismutase, which protects against free radical–mediated degradation of hyaluronic acid, is encoded by chromosome 21[23]. Since superoxide dismutase is overexpressed in trisomy 21 fetuses[24], there may be a decrease in the degradation of hyaluronic acid.

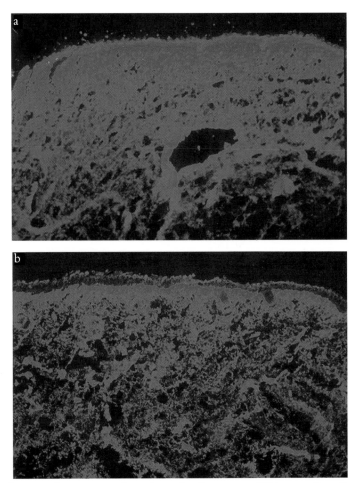

Figure 12 Immunofluorescence detection of collagen type VI in a section through nuchal skin of a fetus with trisomy 21 (a) and in a normal control fetus (b). In trisomy 21, there is intense staining of the extracellular matrix, extending to the dermis–subcutis junction, whereas, in the normal fetus, intense staining is restricted to the upper dermis immediately underlying the basement membrane

In fetuses with trisomy 21, increased amounts of hyaluronic acid may not be restricted to the nuchal skin but are probably found in other tissues and organs contributing to the pathogenesis of other abnormalities. A single chain of hyaluronic acid, through link proteins, is bound to a great number of aggrecan (a protein) monomers to form large aggregates which inhibit cell movement. For example, matrices containing hyaluronan-aggregating proteoglycans inhibit the migration of neural crest cells[25]. This may be the underlying mechanism for Hirschsprung disease, which is associated with trisomy 21 and which is thought to be the consequence of failure of migration of

Table 2 Genetic syndromes associated with increased nuchal translucency, which may be mediated by altered composition of the extracellular matrix

Protein	Gene	Chromosome	Condition
Collagen I, α1 polypeptide	COL1A1	7q	osteogenesis imperfecta II
Collagen I, α2 polypeptide	COL1A2	17q	Ehlers–Danlos syndrome VIIA2 atypical Marfan syndrome
Collagen II, α1 polypeptide	COL2A1	12q	achondrogenesis II Stickler syndrome
Collagen XI, α2 polypeptide	COL11A2	6p 4p	Nance–Sweeney syndrome Stickler syndrome II
Fibroblast growth factor receptor-3	FGFR3	7q	achondroplasia hypochondroplasia thanatophoric dysplasia I and II Crouzon syndrome
Peroxisome biogenesis factor-1	PEX1 ZWS1		Zellweger syndrome

neuroblasts from the neural crest to the bowel segments, a process which normally occurs at 6–12 weeks of gestation.

Another possible mechanism for a link between alterations in the composition of collagen type VI (which is a powerful substrate for cell adhesion) and increased nuchal translucency is impairment in cardiac function or structure. The atrioventricular–septal defects, commonly observed in trisomy 21, may be the consequence of failure of endocardial cushion fusion, due to increased adhesiveness of fibroblasts[26,27].

Altered composition of the extracellular matrix may also be the underlying mechanism for increased fetal nuchal translucency in an expanding number of genetic syndromes (Table 2), which are associated with alterations in collagen metabolism (such as achondrogenesis type II, Nance–Sweeney syndrome, osteogenesis imperfecta type II), abnormalities of fibroblast growth factor receptors (such as achondroplasia and thanatophoric dysplasia) or disturbed metabolism of peroxisome biogenesis factor (such as Zellweger syndrome).

LYMPHATIC VESSEL HYPOPLASIA

In normal embryos, the main lymphatics develop from the venous walls, but they subsequently lose their connections with the veins to form a separate lymphatic system, except for the juguloaxillary sacs, which drain the lymph to the venous system[28]. A possible mechanism for increased translucency is dilatation of the jugular lymphatic sacs, because of developmental delay in the connection with the venous system, or a primary abnormal dilatation or proliferation of the lymphatic channels interfering with a normal flow between the lymphatic and venous systems[29].

A microscopical study, examining the lymphatic vessels in the skin of spontaneously aborted fetuses with cervical cystic hygromas, reported that in non-Turner fetuses there were numerous dilated lymphatic vessels, whereas in fetuses with Turner syndrome there were very few such vessels. In the skin of normal fetuses with no cystic hygromas, lymphatic vessels were evenly distributed[30].

Further support for lymphatic hypoplasia in Turner syndrome has been provided by studies investigating women with ovarian dysgenesis as a result of a 45,XO karyotype; in these cases, lymphangiography revealed hypoplastic lymphatic vessels in the lower limbs, pelvis and retroperitoneal space[31].

Immunohistochemical studies have investigated the distribution of lymphatic vessels in nuchal skin tissue from fetuses with Turner syndrome, compared to fetuses with trisomies 21, 18 and 13, that also had increased nuchal translucency, and chromosomally normal controls[32]. The distribution of vessels was examined using PTN63 (an antibody against 5'nucleotidase, which primarily stains lymphatic vessels, but is also present in large endothelial venules of lymphoid tissues), laminin (which is a major component of basement membranes and therefore highlights large lymphatics and both large and small blood vessels) and FLT-4 (an antibody against the vascular endothelial growth factor receptor-3, whose expression is essentially restricted to lymphatic endothelia during development). Vascular endothelial growth factors (VEGF) play important roles in angiogenesis and vascular development during embryogenesis; these growth factors act through three receptors VEGFR1, VEGFR2 and VEGFR3[33]. In the nuchal skin of normal fetuses and those with trisomies 21, 18 and 13, PTN63-positive, laminin-positive and FLT-4-positive vessels were evenly distributed throughout the dermis and subcutis. In Turner syndrome, there was a chain of large vessels at the border between the dermis and subcutis, which was stained by all three stains. However, in the upper dermis, although there was intense staining with laminin of small and medium-size vessels, there were no PTN63-positive or FLT-4-positive vessels. These findings indicate that, in Turner syndrome, the lymphatic vessels in the upper dermis are hypoplastic (Figure 13). In contrast, the increased nuchal translucency of trisomic fetuses cannot be attributed to lymphatic hypoplasia.

A possible mechanism for hypoplasia of lymphatic vessels in Turner syndrome is deficiency in the tyrosine kinase BMX, whose gene is located on chromosome X. This tyrosine kinase is expressed in the endothelial cells of several human tissues[34] and it is possible that this kinase plays an important role in mediating the effects of the vascular endothelial growth factors for the development of early blood and lymphatic vessels.

Immunohistochemistry and *in situ* hybridization studies examined the distribution of a wide range of proteoglycans in the nuchal skin of chromosomally abnormal fetuses with increased nuchal translucency. Proteoglycans are involved in fluid retention as well as growth and migration of lymphatic vessels. Altered composition of the

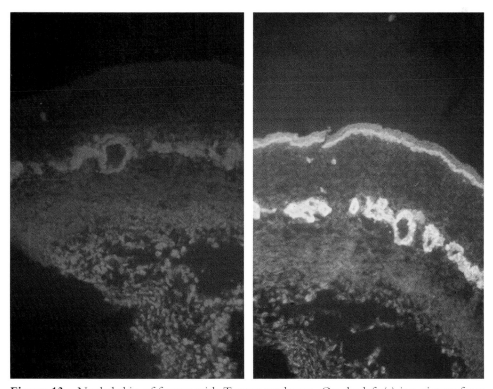

Figure 13 Nuchal skin of fetuses with Turner syndrome. On the left (a) is a picture from single staining with monoclonal PTN63 antibody (red) showing the absence of lymphatic vessels in the upper dermis and a chain of dilated vessels in the junction between the dermis and subcutis. On the right (b) is double staining with both PTN63 and laminin antibodies demonstrating yellow–orange fluorescence in the chain of dilated vessels. Vessels in the upper dermis are only laminin-positive (green)

extracellular matrix may result in abnormal accumulation of fluid, but it can also entrap and inhibit the physiological effects of growth factors on developing blood and lymphatic vessels. The studies demonstrated that, in the skin of fetuses with Turner syndrome, proteoglycan expression was substantially different from normal. In particular, biglycan, which is encoded on chromosome X, was underexpressed and chondroitin-6-sulfate was overexpressed. In fetuses with trisomies 21, 18 or 13, compared to chromosomally normal controls, there was no obvious difference in proteoglycan expression.

ANEMIA AND HYPOPROTEINEMIA

Anemia and hypoproteinemia are implicated in the pathophysiology of both immune and non-immune hydrops fetalis[35–37]. Since trisomy 21 is associated with reduced maternal serum concentration of α-fetoprotein, it is possible that these fetuses are hypoproteinemic (the source of maternal serum α-fetoprotein is the fetus). However, investigation of the α-fetoprotein mRNA gene expression in the liver of fetuses with trisomy 21 showed no significant difference from normal[38].

In a study of 32 fetuses with homozygous α-thalassemia, there was an overall increase in nuchal translucency thickness by about 0.4 mm, compared to normal controls, but this increase was clinically insignificant[39]. This finding indirectly suggests that the increased nuchal translucency in trisomic fetuses cannot be explained by fetal anemia.

CONGENITAL INFECTION

In about 10% of cases of 'unexplained' second- or third-trimester fetal hydrops, there is evidence of recent maternal infection and, in these cases, the fetus is also infected. In a study of 426 pregnancies with increased fetal nuchal translucency and normal karyotype, only 1.5% of the mothers had evidence of recent infection and none of the fetuses was infected[40]. These findings suggest that, in pregnancies with increased fetal nuchal translucency, the prevalence of maternal infection with the TORCH group of organisms is not higher than in the general population. Furthermore, in cases of maternal infection, the presence of increased fetal nuchal translucency does not signify the presence of fetal infection with these organisms. Therefore, increased nuchal translucency in chromosomally normal fetuses need not stimulate the search for maternal infection unless the translucency evolves into second- or third-trimester nuchal edema or generalized hydrops.

In a report of three cases of recent maternal infection with parvovirus B19, fetal hydrops developed at 12 weeks of gestation; in all three cases, the hydrops resolved by 22 weeks and healthy babies were born[41]. The possible mechanism for the transient hydrops is heart failure due to myocardial infection. The alternative of bone marrow suppression, leading to fetal anemia and high-output heart failure, is unlikely because at 12 weeks the main hemopoietic organ in the fetus is the liver rather than the marrow.

REFERENCES

1. Hyett JA, Moscoso G, Nicolaides KH. Abnormalites of the heart and great arteries in first trimester chromosomally abnormal fetuses. *Am J Med Genet* 1997;69:207–16

2. Hyett JA, Moscoso G, Nicolaides KH. Morphometric analysis of the great vessels in early fetal life. *Hum Reprod* 1995;10:3045–8

3. Hyett JA, Moscoso G, Nicolaides KH. Increased nuchal translucency in trisomy 21 fetuses: relation to narrowing of the aortic isthmus. *Hum Reprod* 1995;10:3049–51

4. Snijders RJM, Noble P, Sebire N, Souka A, Nicolaides KH. UK multicentre project on assessment of risk of trisomy 21 by maternal age and fetal nuchal translucency thickness at 10–14 weeks of gestation. *Lancet* 1998;352:343–6

5. Clark EB. Neck web and congenital heart defects: a pathogenic association in 45 X-O Turner syndrome? *Teratology* 1984;29:355–61

6. Miyabara S, Sugihara H, Maehara N, Shouno H, Tasaki H, Yoshida K, Saito N, Kayama F, Ibara S, Suzumori K, Miyabara S. Significance of cardiovascular malformations in cystic hygroma: a new interpretation of the pathogenesis. *Am J Med Genet* 1989;34:489–501

7. Besson WT, Kirby ML, Van Mierop LH, Teabeaut JR. Effects of the size of lesions of the cardiac neural crest at various embryonic ages on incidence and type of cardiac defects. *Circulation* 1986;73:360–4

8. Halford S, Wadey R, Roberts C, Daw SC, Whiting JA, O'Donnell H, Dunham I, Bentley D, Lindsay E, Baldini A, *et al.* Isolation of a putative transcriptional regulator from the region of 22q11 deleted in DiGeorge syndrome, Shprintzen syndrome and familial congenital heart disease. *Hum Mol Genet* 1993;2:2099–107

9. Montenegro N, Matias A, Areias JC, Castedo S, Barros H. Increased fetal nuchal translucency: possible involvement of early cardiac failure. *Ultrasound Obstet Gynecol* 1997;10:265–8

10. Matias A, Gomes C, Flack N, Montenegro N, Nicolaides K. Screening for chromosomal abnormalities at 11–14 weeks: the role of ductus venosus blood flow. *Ultrasound Obstet Gynecol* 1998;12:380–4

11. Huisman TW, Bilardo CM. Transient increase in nuchal translucency thickness and reversed end-diastolic ductus venosus flow in a fetus with trisomy 18. *Ultrasound Obstet Gynecol* 1997;10:397–9

12. Hyett JA, Brizot ML, von Kaisenberg CS, McKie AT, Farzaneh F, Nicolaides KH. Cardiac gene expression of atrial natriuretic peptide and brain natriuretic peptide in trisomic fetuses. *Obstet Gynecol* 1996;87:506–10

13. Tsuchimochi H, Kurimoto F, Ieki K, Koyama H, Takaku F, Kawana M, Kimata S, Yazaki Y. Atrial natriuretic peptide distribution in fetal and failed adult human hearts. *Circulation* 1988;78:920–7

14. Sebire NJ, Snijders RJ, Davenport M, Greenough A, Nicolaides KH. Fetal nuchal translucency thickness at 10–14 weeks' gestation and congenital diaphragmatic hernia. *Obstet Gynecol* 1997;90: 943–6

15. Bronshtein M, Lewit N, Sujov P, Makhoul I, Blazer S. Prenatal diagnosis of congenital diaphragmatic hernia: timing of visceral herniation and outcome. *Prenat Diagn* 1995;15:695–8

16. von Kaisenberg CS, Brand-Saberi B, Christ B, Vallian S, Farzaneh F, Nicolaides KH. Collagen type VI gene expression in the skin of trisomy 21 fetuses. *Obstet Gynecol* 1998;91:319–23

17. von Kaisenberg CS, Krenn V, Ludwig M, Nicolaides KH, Brand-Saberi B. Morphological classification of nuchal skin in fetuses with trisomy 21, 18 and 13 at 12–18 weeks and in a trisomy 16 mouse. *Anat Embryol* 1998;197:105–24

18. Golaz J, Charnay Y, Vallet P, Bouras C. Alzheimer's disease and Down's syndrome. Some recent etiopathogenic data. *Encephale* 1991;17:29–31

19. Sumarsono SH, Wilson TJ, Tymms MJ, Venter DJ, Corrick CM, Kola R *et al.* Down's syndrome-like skeletal abnormalities in Ets2 transgenic mice. *Nature* 1996;379:534–7

20. McDevitt CA, Marcelino J, Tucker L. Interaction of intact type VI collagen with hyaluronan. *FEBS Lett* 1991;294:167–70

21. Engström-Laurent A. Changes in hyaluronan concentration in tissue and body fluids in disease states. *Ciba Found Symp* 1989;143:233–47

22. Hay E. *Cell Biology of Extracellular Matrix*, 2nd edn. New York: Plenum Press, 1991:163

23. De La Torre R, Casado A, Lopez-Fernandez E, Carrascosa D, Ramirez V, Saez J. Overexpression of copper-zinc superoxide dismutase in trisomy 21. *Experientia* 1996;52:871–3

24. Aliakbar S, Brown PR, Bidwell D, Nicolaides KH. Human erythrocyte superoxide dismutase in adults, neonates, and normal, hypoxaemic, anaemic, and chromosomally abnormal fetuses. *Clin Biochem* 1993;26:109–15

25. Perris R, Johansson S. Inhibition of neural crest cell migration by aggregating chondroitin sulfate proteoglycans is mediated by their hyaluronan-binding region. *Dev Biol* 1990;137:1–12

26. Kurnit DM, Aldridge JF, Matsouka R, Matthyse S. Increased adhesiveness of trisomy 21 cells and atrioventricular canal malformations in Down syndrome: a stochastic model. *Am J Med Genet* 1985;30:385–99

27. Kurnit DM, Layton WM, Matthyse S. Genetics, chance and morphogenesis. In Epstein CJ, ed. *Morphogenesis of Down syndrome*. New York: Wiley Liss, 1987:19–41

28. van der Putte SCJ, van Limborogh J. The embryonic development of the main lymphatics in man. *Acta Morphol Neerl-Scand* 1980;8:323–35

29. van der Putte SCJ. Lymphatic malformation in human fetuses. *Virchows Arch[A]* 1977;376:233–46

30. Chitayat D, Kalousek DK, Bamforth JS. Lymphatic abnormalities in fetuses with posterior cervical cystic hygroma. *Am J Med Genet* 1989;33:352–6

31. Vittay P, Bosze P, Gaal M, Laszlo J. Lymph vessel defects in patients with ovarian dysgenesis. *Clin Genet* 1980;18:387–91

32. von Kaisenberg CS, Nicolaides KH, Brand-Saberi B. Lymphatic vessel hypoplasia in fetuses with Turner syndrome. *Hum Reprod* 1999;14:823–6

33. Joukov V, Pajusola K, Kaipainen A, Chilov D, Lahtinen I, Kukk E, Saksela O, Kalkkinen N, Alitalo K. A novel vascular endothelial growth factor, VEGF-C, is a ligand for the Flt4 (VEGFR-3) and KDR (VEGFR-2) receptor tyrosine kinases. *EMBO J* 1996;15:290–8

34. Tamagnone L, Lahtinen I, Mustonen T, Virtaneva K, Francis F, Muscatelli F, Alitalo R, Smith CIE, Larsson C, Alitalo K. BMX, a novel nonreceptor tyrosine kinase gene of the BTK/ITK/TEC/TXK family located in chromosome Xp22.2. *Oncogene* 1994;9:3683–8

35. Nicolaides KH. Warens hemoglobin level to the development of hydrops in rhesus isoimmunization. *Am J Obstet Gynecol* 1985;152:341–4

36. Nicolaides KH, Rodeck CH, Lange I, Watson J, Gosden CM, Millar D, Mibashan RS, Moniz C, Morgan-Capner P, Campbell S. Fetoscopy in the assessment of unexplained fetal hydrops. *Br J Obstet Gynaecol* 1985;92:671–9

37. Nicolaides KH, Rodeck CH, Millar DS, Mibashan RS. Fetal haematology in rhesus isoimmunisation. *Br Med J* 1985;1:661–3

38. Brizot ML, McKie AT, von Kaisenberg CS, Farzaneh F, Nicolaides KH. Fetal hepatic AFP mRNA expression in fetuses with trisomy 21 and trisomy 18 at 12–15 weeks of gestation. *Early Hum Dev* 1996;44:155–9

39. Lam YH, Tang MH, Lee CP, Tse HY. Nuchal translucency in fetuses affected by homozygous α-thalassemia-1 at 12–13 weeks of gestation. *Ultrasound Obstet Gynecol* 1999;13:238–40

40. Sebire NJ, Bianco D, Snijders RJM, Zuckerman M, Nicolaides KH. Increased fetal nuchal translucency thickness at 10–14 weeks: is screening for maternal-fetal infection necessary? *Br J Obstet Gynaecol* 1997;104:212–15

41. Petrikovsky BM, Baker D, Schneider E. Fetal hydrops secondary to human parvovirus infection in early pregnancy. *Prenat Diagn* 1996;16:342–4

4

Diagnosis of fetal abnormalities at the 11–14-week scan

The early pregnancy scan was initially introduced with the primary intention of measuring the fetal crown–rump length to achieve accurate pregnancy dating. During the last decade, however, improvement in the resolution of ultrasound machines has made it possible to describe the normal anatomy of the fetus and diagnose or suspect the presence of a wide range of fetal defects in the first trimester of pregnancy. In some conditions, the sonographic features are similar to those described in the second and third trimesters of pregnancy, but in others there are characteristic sonographic features confined to the first trimester.

NORMAL FIRST-TRIMESTER ULTRASOUND FINDINGS

'Normal human embryogenesis is a stereotyped sequence with little statistical variation, but menstrual data in individual cases may be unreliable in dating this sequence'[1]. An embryo of 10 postmenstrual weeks is less than half the length of an adult thumb, but already possesses several thousand named structures, practically any of which may be subject to developmental deviations[2]. Thus, the embryonic period proper is of particular importance because the majority of congenital anomalies make their appearance during that time[2]. These statements from embryological investigations have become highly relevant for those involved in first-trimester ultrasound scanning.

The term sonoembryology[3] designates the description of the embryonic anatomy, the normal anatomic relations and the development of abnormalities as visualized by ultrasound. To confirm the presence of normal anatomy or to make the diagnosis of an anomaly, we need knowledge of the normal embryonic development, including the appearance of the normal embryo. This section is based on data from sonoembryological and embryological studies[4–13]. For the ultrasound studies, 7.5-MHz transducers were used.

4 weeks

At 4 weeks and 3 days, a tiny gestational sac becomes visible within the decidua.

5 weeks

The yolk sac is first visible at 5 weeks and it is always present by 5 weeks and 4 days. There are lacunary structures at the site of implantation. The embryonic pole appears adjacent to the yolk sac, soon showing cardiac activity. Since the connecting stalk is short, the embryonic pole is found near the wall. At the end of week 5, the heart rate is about 100 bpm.

6 weeks (crown–rump length 4–8 mm)

The embryonic pole, yolk sac and heart activity are now always present. The heart rate increases to 130 bpm. At the end of week 6, the first sign of the rhombencephalic cavity appears as a tiny hypoechogenic area in the cranial pole of the embryo. The amniotic cavity can be seen surrounded by a thin membrane around the embryo.

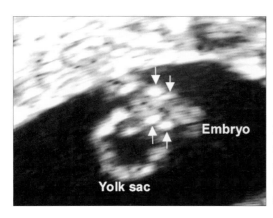

Figure 1 Embryo at 6 weeks (crown–rump length 5 mm). Coronal section with arrows pointing to the ventricular and atrial parts of the primitive heart. The yolk sac lies adjacent to the embryo

7 weeks (crown–rump length 9–14 mm)

External form

The embryonic body appears as a triangle in the sagittal section. The sides consist of (1) the back, (2) the roof of the rhombencephalon, and (3) the frontal part of the head, the base of the umbilical cord, and the embryonic tail. The embryonic body is slender in the coronal plane. The limbs are short, paddle-shaped outgrowths.

Central nervous system

The hypoechogenic brain cavities can be identified, including the separated cerebral hemispheres. The lateral ventricles are shaped like small, round vesicles. The cavity of the diencephalon (future third ventricle) runs posteriorly. In the smallest embryos, the medial telencephalon forms a continuous cavity between the lateral ventricles. The future foramina of Monro are wide during week 7. In the sagittal plane, the height of the cavity of the diencephalon is slightly greater than that of the mesencephalon (future Sylvian aqueduct). Thus, the wide border between the cavities of the diencephalon and the mesencephalon is indicated. The curved tube-like mesencephalic cavity lies anteriorly, its rostral part pointing caudally. It straightens considerably during the following weeks. By week 8, it is regularly identified. The relatively broad and shallow

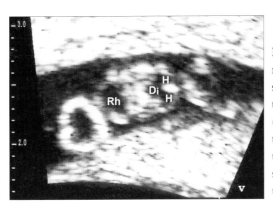

Figure 2 Embryo at 7⁺² weeks (crown–rump length 12 mm). Oblique transverse section through the head demonstrating the rhombencephalon (Rh), diencephalon (Di) and hemispheres (H). The connections between the lateral ventricles and third ventricle (foramina of Monro) are still wide. The echogenic ring to the left is the yolk sac

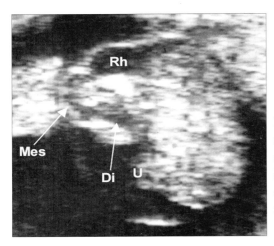

Figure 3 Embryo at 7⁺⁵ weeks (crown–rump length 14 mm). Sagittal section through the 'triangular' body demonstrating the shallow cavity of the rhombencephalon (Rh), the curved tube-like mesencephalon (Mes), the diencephalon (Di) and the umbilical cord (U)

rhombencephalic cavity is always visible from 7 weeks onwards. It then has a well-defined rhombic shape in the cranial pole of the embryo.

Heart

The heart can be recognized as a beating, large and bright structure below the embryonic head at 7 weeks. The heart rate increases from 130 bpm to 160 bpm. Details of the heart anatomy are not visible, but the atrial and ventricular compartments can sometimes be distinguished by the reciprocal movements of the walls.

Intestinal tract

The short umbilical cord shows a large celomic cavity at its insertion, where the primary intestinal loop can be identified. The first sign of herniation of the gut occurs during week 7 as a thickening of the cord and showing a slight echogenic area at the abdominal insertion. Within a few days, this echogenic structure becomes more distinct.

Extra-embryonic structures

The amniotic cavity becomes visible at the beginning of week 7. The mean diameter of the amniotic cavity is almost the same as the corresponding crown–rump length.

8 weeks (crown–rump length 15–22 mm)

External form

The body gradually grows thicker and becomes cuboidal. At the end of the week, the elbows become obvious, the hands angle from the sagittal plane and the fingers are distinguishable.

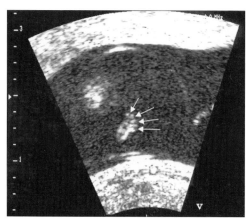

Figure 4 Embryo at 8^{+3} weeks (crown–rump length 18 mm). The fingers (arrows) are visible

Central nervous system

The brain cavities are easily seen as large 'holes' in the embryonic head. The hemispheres enlarge, developing via thick round slices originating antero-caudally from the third ventricle into a crescent shape. The choroid plexus in the lateral ventricles becomes visible as tiny echogenic areas. The future foramina of Monro become more accentuated during week 8. The third ventricle is still relatively wide, as is the mesencephalic cavity. At this stage, the mesencephalon lies at the top of the head. The increased growth of the rostral brain structures and the deepening of the pontine flexure leads to the deflection of the brain. The rhombencephalic cavity (future fourth ventricle) has a pyramid-like shape with the central deepening of the pontine flexure as the peak of the pyramid. The first signs of the bilateral choroid plexuses are lateral echogenic areas originating near the branches of the medulla oblongata caudal to the lateral recesses. Within a short time, the choroid plexuses traverse the roof of the fourth ventricle, meeting in the mid-line and dividing the roof into two portions, about two-thirds are located rostrally and one-third caudally. In the sagittal section, the choroid plexuses are identified as an echogenic fold of the roof.

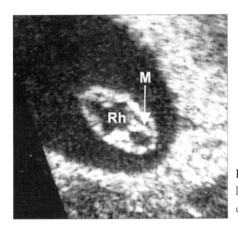

Figure 5 Embryo at 8^{+1} weeks (crown–rump length 17 mm). Section through the rhombencephalon (Rh) and mesencephalon (arrow, M)

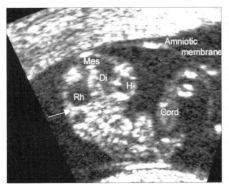

Figure 6 Embryo at 8^{+5} weeks (crown–rump length 18 mm). Slightly parasagittal section demonstrating the ventricle of one hemisphere (H) leading through the foramen of Monro into the third ventricle, which is the cavity of the diencephalon (Di). The wide mesencephalic cavity (Mes) lies at the top of the head and the cavity of the rhombencephalon lies posteriorly. The arrow points at the choroid plexus of the rhombencephalon

Heart

The heart rate has increased to 160 bpm. Occasionally it is possible to identify the atrial and ventricular walls moving reciprocally as early as at the end of week 8. The atrial compartment appears wider than the ventricular compartment, and the heart covers about 50% of the transverse thoracic area. A kind of four-chamber view of the heart can then be obtained, where the atrial compartment is wider than the ventricular part.

Intestinal tract

There is no sign of the stomach during week 7. In some cases, it is possible to recognize the fluid-filled stomach as a small hypoechogenic area on the left side of the upper abdomen below the heart at the end of week 8.

9 weeks (crown–rump length 23–31 mm)

External form

The body develops an ellipsoid shape with a large head. The soles of the feet touch in the mid-line at the end of the week. At the same time, it is possible to obtain acceptable images of the profile; thus, it should be possible to examine the mouth. The ventral body wall is well defined.

Central nervous system

The lateral ventricles are always visible. They are best seen in the parasagittal plane, where the C-shape becomes apparent. The cortex is smooth and hypoechogenic. The bright choroid plexuses of the lateral ventricles are regularly detectable at 9 weeks 4 days. They show rapid growth, similar to the hemispheres, and soon fill most of the ventricular cavities. The width of the diencephalic cavity narrows gradually, while the

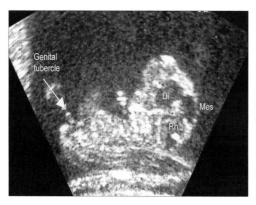

Figure 7 Embryo at 9^{+4} weeks (crown–rump length 28 mm). Sagittal section demonstrating the relatively large head and the cavities of the diencephalon (Di), mesencephalon (Mes) and rhombencephalon (Rh). The arrow points at the genital tubercle, but at this stage it is not possible to differentiate between male and female gender

width of the mesencephalon remains wide. A distinct border ('isthmus prosencephali') has developed between the cavity of the mesencephalon and the third ventricle. The wall of the diencephalon, initially very thin, thickens considerably starting from week 8 to 9. The isthmus rhombencephali is always distinct. The cavity of the mesencephalon remains relatively large, especially the posterior part. The height and the width are about the same size. During weeks 8 and 9, the rhombic fossa becomes deeper due to the progressive flexure of the pons. The lateral corners of the rhombencephalic cavity, called the lateral recesses, are easily identified at weeks 7 and 8. During this period, the distance between these recesses increases (rhombencephalon width). Later, during weeks 9 and 10, the lateral recesses often become covered by the enlarging cerebellar hemispheres. Thus, only the central part of the hypoechogenic fourth ventricle, which is divided by the choroid plexuses, is visible. The choroid plexuses of the fourth ventricle are bright landmarks, dividing the ventricle into rostral and caudal compartments. The cerebellar hemispheres are easily detectable. The primordia of cerebellar hemispheres are clearly separated in the mid-line during the embryonic period.

Heart

During week 9, the heart rate reaches a maximum of mean 175 bpm.

Intestinal tract

From 8 weeks 3 days to 10 weeks 4 days of gestational age, all embryos have herniation of the midgut, most distinctive during weeks 9 and 10. At this stage, the midgut herniation presents as a large hyperechogenic mass. The stomach can be detected in 75% of the embryos before 10 weeks.

Postembryonic period, weeks 10 and 11 (crown–rump length 32–54 mm)

External form

The human features of the fetus become clearer. The fetal body elongates, the arms and the legs develop into upper and lower arms and legs, the hands and fingers and the feet and toes. In the largest fetuses, the soles of the feet rotate from the sagittal plane. The head is still relatively large with a prominent forehead and a flat occiput. The future skull can be distinguished; ossification starts at about 11 weeks with the occipital bone[14].

Central nervous system

The thick crescent-shaped lateral ventricles fill the anterior part of the head and conceal the diencephalic cavity. The thickness of the cortex is about 1 mm at the end of the first trimester. The diencephalon lies between the hemispheres, and the mesencephalon gradually moves towards the center of the head. After an initial increase, the width of the third ventricle becomes narrow towards the end of the first trimester. The cerebellar hemispheres seem to meet in the mid-line during weeks 11–12. After 10 weeks 3 days, the choroid plexuses of the fourth ventricle can always be visualized. The distance between the choroid plexuses and the cerebellum becomes shorter during weeks 9–11 because of cerebellar growth. The onset of ossification of the spine occurs at the end of the first trimester.

Heart

At 10 weeks, the moving valves and the interventricular septum can be identified. The heart rate slows down to 165 bpm at the end of week 11. The ventricles, atria, septa, valves, veins and outflow tracts become identifiable.

Intestinal tract

Midgut herniation has its maximal extension at the beginning of week 10 and returns into the abdominal cavity during weeks 10–11. The gut retracts into the abdominal cavity between 10 weeks 4 days and 11 weeks 5 days. Fetuses which are older than 11 weeks 5 days usually do not demonstrate any sign of the herniation. The esophagus can be identified as an echogenic double line anterior to the aorta, leading into the stomach. The stomach is visible in all specimens before 11 completed weeks.

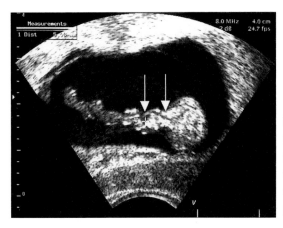

Figure 8 Embryo at 10 weeks (crown–rump length 32 mm). Horizontal section through the abdomen demonstrating the umbilical cord. The arrows show the extension of the physiological midgut herniation

Fetal growth from 7 to 12 weeks

The longitudinal measurements of the biparietal diameter, occipito-frontal diameter, mean abdominal diameter, crown–rump length, amniotic cavity diameter and chorionic cavity diameter show a high degree of uniformity with virtually the same growth velocities. The yolk sac demonstrates uniform growth until week 10 only.

ABNORMAL ULTRASOUND FINDINGS

CENTRAL NERVOUS SYSTEM DEFECTS

Acrania / exencephaly / anencephaly

Prenatal ultrasonographic diagnosis of anencephaly during the second and third trimesters of pregnancy is based on the demonstration of an absent cranial vault and cerebral hemispheres[15]. Animal studies have shown that, in the absence of the cranial vault, there is progressive degeneration of the exposed cerebral tissue to anencephaly[16].

In normal human fetuses, there is histological evidence that the onset of ossification of the cranial vault is at 10 weeks of gestation[17] and that, ultrasonographically by 11 weeks, there is hyperechogenicity of the skull in comparison to the underlying tissues[18]. Ultrasound reports have demonstrated that in the human, as in animal studies, there is progression from acrania to exencephaly and finally anencephaly (Table 1)[19–23]. In the first trimester, the pathognomonic feature is acrania, the brain being either entirely normal or at varying degrees of distortion and disruption.

Goldstein *et al.* reported the difficulties with early diagnosis of anencephaly; the 12-week scan showed no defects but repeat examination at 26 weeks demonstrated anencephaly[24]. Rottem *et al.* reported a fetus at 9 weeks with an abnormal shape of the cephalic pole and cervical spine; at 11 weeks, the diagnosis of anencephaly and open

Table 1 Case reports on the prenatal diagnosis of anencephaly at 11–14 weeks of gestation

Author	*Case*	*Gestation* (weeks)	*Ultrasound findings*
Schmidt and Kubli 1982[19]	1	13	anencephaly
Johnson *et al.* 1985[20]	2	11	anencephaly
Rottem *et al.* 1989[21]	3	9	abnormal cephalic pole
		11	anencephaly
Kennedy *et al.* 1990[22]	4	10	exencephaly
Bronshtein and Ornoy 1991[23]	5	9	normal
		11	normal
		12	acrania
		14	anencephaly

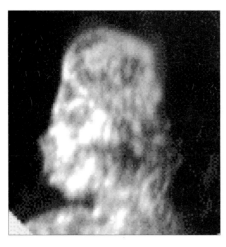

Figure 9 Acrania in an 11-week fetus

cervical spina bifida was made[21]. Kennedy *et al.* described a case of acrania at 10 weeks in which the brain was of normal volume but appeared echogenic and disorganized; at 14 weeks, the fragmented and degenerating brain was visualized[22]. Bronshtein and Ornoy reported a case with no abnormal findings at 9 and 11 weeks, but at 12 weeks there was acrania and at 14 weeks there was anencephaly[23].

Screening studies

In an ultrasound screening study of 622 high-risk pregnancies at 10–13 weeks and 16–18 weeks of gestation, all three fetuses with acrania/anencephaly were correctly identified at the first scan[25]. Another screening study examined 3991 patients by ultrasound at 11–14 weeks and again at 18–20 weeks; there were two cases of exencephaly (one associated with spina bifida and another with iniencephaly) and they were both diagnosed at the early scan[26]. Two screening studies for chromosomal abnormalities by fetal nuchal translucency at 10–14 weeks in a total of 6861 pregnancies correctly diagnosed all seven cases of anencephaly in the first-trimester scan[27,28].

In a multicenter study of screening for chromosomal abnormalities, by assessment of fetal nuchal translucency thickness at 10–14 weeks of gestation, there were 53 435 singleton and 901 twin pregnancies[29]. There were 47 fetuses with anencephaly, including three from twin pregnancies. The diagnosis of anencephaly was made at the early scan in 39 cases and at the 16–22-week scan in a further eight cases. During the first phase of the study, 34 830 fetuses were examined. In this group, there were 31 cases of anencephaly but the diagnosis was made at the early scan in only 23 (74%) of the cases[29]. Subsequently, the sonographers from the participating centers were informed of the different diagnostic features of anencephaly in the first compared to the second trimester and they were instructed to specifically look for and record the presence or absence of acrania at the early scan. In the second phase of the study, 20 407 fetuses were examined and all 16 cases of anencephaly were diagnosed at the early scan[29].

These findings demonstrate that anencephaly can be reliably diagnosed at the routine 11–14-week ultrasound scan, provided the sonographic features for this condition are specifically searched for.

Encephalocele

This is a cranial defect with protrusion of meninges (meningocele) and brain (encephalocele). In about 75% of cases, the lesion is occipital but alternative sites include the frontoethmoidal and parietal regions. It is often associated with microcephaly, hydrocephaly, spina bifida and Meckel–Gruber syndrome.

A prerequisite for the diagnosis of encephalocele (in contrast to nuchal cystic hygroma) is the demonstration of an associated bony defect in the skull and, therefore, the diagnosis may not be possible before the onset of cranial ossification at about 10 weeks of gestation. However, van Zalen-Sprock et al. have reported that, at least in some cases, the first sign for possible encephalocele is enlargement of the rhombencephalic cavity from about 9 weeks[30].

Bronshtein and Zimmer described a case of occipital encephalocele that was first seen at 13 weeks as an empty occipital sac measuring 8×9 mm[31]. At 14 weeks, the sac remained of the same size and was filled with brain tissue. At 15 and 16 weeks, repeated examinations demonstrated complete resolution of the defect and the maternal serum

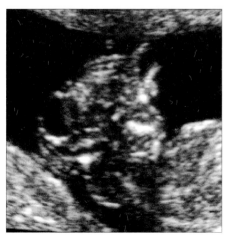

Figure 10   Encephalocele in a 12-week fetus

α-fetoprotein was normal. At 19 weeks, there was recurrence of the encephalocele and this persisted until 24 weeks when the pregnancy was terminated; pathological examination confirmed the diagnosis of encephalocele.

van Zalen-Sprock et al. described a fetus at 11 weeks of gestation with two translucent areas in the occipital region[32]. A repeat scan at 13 weeks demonstrated a bony defect and protrusion of the brain. The diagnosis of occipital encephalocele was made and this was confirmed by pathological examination after termination of the pregnancy.

Meckel–Gruber syndrome

This is a lethal, autosomal recessive condition characterized by the triad of encephalocele, bilateral polycystic kidneys and polydactyly.

Pachi et al. described the sonographic features of the syndrome in a high-risk pregnancy at 13 weeks of gestation[33]. There was an occipital bony defect accompanied by encephalocele and abnormally enlarged kidneys. Pathological examination, after termination at 13 weeks, detected all three features of the syndrome. Sepulveda et al. examined nine high-risk pregnancies at 11–13 weeks and correctly diagnosed the four affected fetuses by the presence of the characteristic triad of the syndrome[34]. Similarly, van Zalen-Sprock et al. examined five high-risk pregnancies and correctly identified the three affected fetuses at 11–14 weeks[30].

Screening studies

An ultrasound screening study for fetal abnormalities at 12–14 weeks of gestation, involving 1632 pregnancies correctly identified the one case of Meckel–Gruber syndrome; there was an occipital bony defect with a small encephalocele at 12 weeks and enlarged cystic kidneys at 13 weeks[35]. The parents chose to continue with the pregnancy and at 15 weeks there was enlargement of the encephalocele. Serial scans from 18 weeks demonstrated the presence of anhydramnios, making visualization of the fetal abnormalities difficult. The diagnosis was confirmed after delivery at 37 weeks and neonatal death[36]. Sepulveda et al. detected the triad of the syndrome in a 13-week fetus during screening for chromosomal abnormalities by measurement of fetal nuchal translucency thickness in 21 477 pregnancies[34].

These findings suggest that the phenotypic expression of the syndrome is evident from at least 11 weeks of gestation. Consequently, all affected cases could potentially be diagnosed by the early scan, provided that systematic examination of both the skull/brain and the renal fossae is carried out routinely. Indeed, the diagnosis is likely to

·be easier at 11–14 weeks, when the amniotic fluid is normal, than during the second trimester when the presence of the associated oligohydramnios could easily cause encephalocele and certainly polydactyly to be missed. Additionally, at 11–14 weeks, the fingers are easier to examine because they are invariably extended, whereas in the second trimester the hands are often clenched.

Hydrocephalus

Congenital hydrocephalus has a birth prevalence of about 2 per 1000. Although the underlying cause may be chromosomal abnormalities, genetic syndromes, fetal infection or brain hemorrhage, many cases have no clear-cut etiology and are probably due to a combination of genetic and environmental factors. Antenatal sonographic diagnosis is based on the demonstration of dilated lateral cerebral ventricles.

In normal fetuses, the outline of the lateral ventricles, the echogenic choroid plexi and the mid-line echo are visible by ultrasound from 9 weeks of gestation; at 10–11 weeks, the third and fourth ventricles become visible and, at 12 weeks, the cerebellum and thalamii can be seen[18,37]. The transverse diameter of the choroid plexus increases from 2 mm at 10 weeks to about 5 mm at 13 weeks[7]. The lateral ventricle diameter to hemisphere diameter ratio decreases with gestation from 72% at 12 weeks, 67% at 13 weeks and 61% at 14 weeks[38]. The transverse cerebellar diameter increases linearly with gestation from about 6 mm at 10 weeks to 12 mm at 14 weeks[7,10].

Screening studies

Ventriculomegaly usually develops after the 14th week of gestation. In a screening study involving ultrasound examinations at 11–14 weeks of gestation and again at 18–20 weeks in 3991 patients, there were eight cases of ventriculomegaly (two were associated with spina bifida); only two were diagnosed at the early scan and the other six at 18–20 weeks[26].

Dandy–Walker malformation

This condition, which complicates about 10% of cases with hydrocephalus, is characterized by complete or partial absence of the cerebellar vermis and cystic dilatation of the fourth ventricle. The Dandy–Walker complex is a non-specific end-point of chromosomal abnormalities (usually trisomy 18 or 13 and triploidy), more than 50 genetic syndromes, congenital infection or teratogens such as warfarin, but it can also be an isolated finding.

Ulm *et al.* reported a 14-week fetus with an apparently isolated Dandy–Walker malformation but fetal karyotyping demonstrated triploidy[39].

Screening studies

In a screening study involving ultrasound examinations at 11–14 weeks of gestation and again at 18–20 weeks in 3991 patients, there was one case of the Dandy–Walker malformation and this was not diagnosed in the first-trimester scan[26]. In another screening study for chromosomal abnormalities by fetal nuchal translucency in 1473 pregnancies, there was one case of Dandy–Walker malformation and this was correctly diagnosed in the first-trimester scan[27].

Hydranencephaly

This is a lethal, sporadic condition characterized by absence of the cerebral hemispheres with preservation of the mid-brain and cerebellum. It is thought to result from wide-spread vascular occlusion of the internal carotid arteries or their branches, prolonged severe hydrocephalus, an overwhelming infection, or defects in embryogenesis. About 1% of infants thought to have hydrocephalus are later found to have hydranencephaly.

Lin *et al.* reported a 12-week fetus with a large head, small hemispheres and a fluid-filled intracranial cavity with no mid-line echo[40]. A repeat scan at 18 weeks demonstrated a cystic fetal head with no cerebral hemispheres and falx; the brain could be seen protruding into the cystic cavity. Unlike alobar holoprosencephaly, there was no rim of cortex present. The pregnancy was terminated and pathological examination confirmed the diagnosis.

Holoprosencephaly

Holoprosencephaly, with a birth prevalence of about 1 in 10 000, is characterized by a spectrum of cerebral abnormalities resulting from incomplete cleavage of the forebrain. There are three types according to the degree of forebrain cleavage. The alobar type, which is the most severe, is characterized by a monoventricular cavity and fusion of the thalami. In the semilobar type, there is partial segmentation of the ventricles and cerebral hemispheres posteriorly with incomplete fusion of the thalami. In lobar holoprosencephaly, there is normal separation of the ventricles and thalami but absence of the septum pellucidum. The first two types are often accompanied by facial abnormalities.

Toth *et al.* observed a floating membranous structure in place of the skull of an 11-week fetus[41]. At 12 weeks, they noted acrania and a floating, balloon-like, membranous brain substance. At 16 weeks, the diagnosis of acrania and holoprosencephaly with cyclops was made and these findings were confirmed at postmortem examination after termination at 18 weeks[41]. Bronshtein and Weiner described a case of alobar holoprosencephaly during routine ultrasound examination at 14 weeks; there were a single cerebral ventricle, fused thalami and a crescent-shaped frontal cortex[42]. The fetal karyotype was normal. Gonzalez-Gomez *et al.* described a 10-week fetus with a single ventricular cavity, absence of the orbits and mid-facial cleft[43]. The karyotype was normal. Pathological examination after termination at 11 weeks demonstrated alobar holoprosencephaly, anophthalmia, arrhinia and facial cleft[43]. Sakala and Gaio diagnosed alobar holoprosencephaly in a 13-week fetus with absent falx, large single ventricle and fused thalami; the karyotype was 69,XXY[44]. Turner *et al.* reported a case of alobar holoprosencephaly (single ventricle and fused thalami), exomphalos and increased nuchal translucency at 10 weeks; the karyotype was trisomy 18[45]. Wong *et al.* reported three cases of alobar holoprocencephaly (single ventricle and fused thalami) at 10–13 weeks; there was one case each of trisomy 18, triploidy and mosaic 18p deletion and duplication[46].

Snijders *et al.* reported on the sonographic features of 46 trisomy 13 fetuses at 10–14 weeks of gestation[47]. In 76% there was increased nuchal translucency thickness, 64% were tachycardic, 24% had holoprosencephaly and 10% had exomphalos. There was no significant difference in nuchal translucency thickness between those with and those without holoprosencephaly or exomphalos[47].

Screening studies

In a screening study involving ultrasound examinations at 11–14 weeks of gestation and again at 18–20 weeks in 3991 patients, there was one case of holoprosencephaly and this was not diagnosed in the first-trimester scan[26]. Another screening study for fetal abnormalities at 12–14 weeks of gestation, involving 1632 pregnancies, correctly identified the one case of holoprosencephaly[35].

Iniencephaly

This is a rare malformation of unknown etiology, characterized by cervical dysraphism and occipital (inion) defect with or without an encephalocele.

Sherer *et al.* reported the diagnosis of iniencephaly in a 13-week fetus; there was acrania, persistently hyperextended head and spinal dysraphism[48]. After termination, pathological examination demonstrated complete craniorachischisis with hyper-extended cervical vertebrae.

Spina bifida

In spina bifida, there is failure of closure of the neural tube, which normally occurs by the 6th week of gestation. In the spine of normal fetuses, there are three ossification centers, two pedicles and the spinal body, and these are present from the 10th week of gestation, allowing ultrasonographic visualization of the neural canal from this gestation. Braithwaite *et al.* assessed the fetal anatomy at 12–13 weeks of gestation, by a combination of transabdominal and transvaginal sonography, and they reported successful examination of the vertebrae and overlying skin in both the transverse and coronal planes in all cases[49].

In the 1980s, the main method of screening for open spina bifida was by maternal serum α-fetoprotein at around 16 weeks of gestation and the method of diagnosis was amniocentesis and measurement of amniotic fluid α-fetoprotein and acetyl cholinesterase. Although it was possible to diagnose the condition by ultrasonographic examination of the spine[50], the sensitivity of this test was low[51]. However, the observation, that spina bifida was associated with scalloping of the frontal bones (the 'lemon' sign) (Figure 11), and caudal displacement of the cerebellum (the 'banana' sign)[52], has led to the replacement of biochemical assessment with ultrasonography, both for screening and for diagnosis of this abnormality.

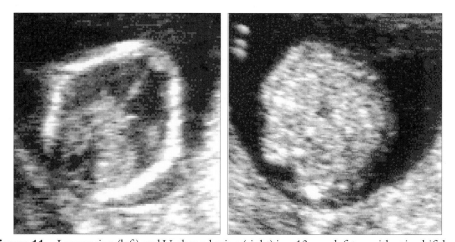

Figure 11   Lemon sign (left) and U-shaped spine (right) in a 13-week fetus with spina bifida

In the 1990s, improvements in the quality of ultrasound equipment have led to the diagnosis of spina bifida during the first trimester of pregnancy. Blumenfeld *et al.* described the evolution of the cranial and cerebellar signs of spina bifida in an affected fetus that was scanned at 10, 12 and 15 weeks of gestation[53]. In the first scan, there was a sacral irregularity but the cerebellum appeared normal; at 12 weeks, the banana sign was detected and, at 15 weeks, when the diagnosis of sacral meningocele was made, the lemon sign was identified. Sebire *et al.* described that, in three cases of lumbosacral spina bifida diagnosed at 12–14 weeks of gestation, there was an associated lemon sign[54]. Similarly, Bernard and colleagues reported the diagnosis of spina bifida in a 12-week fetus with narrowing of the frontal bones and flattening of the occiput[55].

These findings demonstrate that, at least in some cases of spina bifida, the characteristic lemon and banana signs are present from the first trimester of pregnancy. However, the prevalence of these signs at the 11–14-week scan remains to be determined.

Screening studies

In a screening study involving ultrasound examinations at 11–14 weeks of gestation and 18–20 weeks in 3991 patients, there were six cases of spina bifida (including one with associated exencephaly) and five of these were diagnosed at the early scan[26]. In two other screening studies involving 1632 pregnancies at 12–14 weeks[35] and 1473 pregnancies at 10–14 weeks[27], respectively, there were two cases of spina bifida (one in each) and these were not diagnosed in the first-trimester scan.

CARDIAC DEFECTS

Abnormalities of the heart and great arteries are the most common congenital defects and the birth prevalence is 5–10 per 1000. In general, about half are either lethal or require surgery and half are asymptomatic. The first two groups are referred to as major. Specialist echocardiography at around 20 weeks of gestation can identify most of the major cardiac defects, but the main challenge in prenatal diagnosis is to identify the high-risk group for referral to specialist centers. Currently, screening is based on examination of the four-chamber view of the heart at the 20-week scan, but this identifies only 26% of the major cardiac defects[56].

Examination of the four-chamber view of the heart can now be carried out at the 11–14-week scan (Table 2)[57–60]. At 12–13 weeks of gestation, the four-chamber view can be examined successfully by transabdominal ultrasound in 76% of the cases and transvaginally in 95%[49]. Bronshtein *et al.* reported that the diameters of the two ventricles were similar and increased linearly with gestation from about 1.5 mm at 11 weeks

Table 2 Studies reporting on the proportion of cases where the four-chamber view of the heart was successfully visualized by ultrasonography at 10–14 weeks of gestation

Author	10 weeks	11 weeks	12 weeks	13 and 14 weeks
Dolkart & Reimers 1991[57]	0/8	3/10 (30%)	9/10 (90%)	24/24 (100%)
Bronshtein et al. 1992[58]	—	3/18 (16%)	9/25 (36%)	66/72 (90%)
Johnson et al. 1992[59]	7/26 (27%)	19/33 (58%)	36/51 (71%)	73/100 (73%)
Gembruch et al. 1993[60]	—	12/15 (80%)	28/30 (93%)	66/66 (100%)

to 3 mm at 14 weeks; the diameter of the heart was about one-third that of the chest and the ratio did not change with gestation[58]. In contrast, Blaas et al. examined the ratio of the heart diameter to that of the abdomen and reported a decrease with gestation from 51% at 8 weeks to 42% at 12 weeks[11].

Dolkart and Reimers reported that the earliest defined cardiac structures visible were the mitral and tricuspid valves; at 10 weeks, they were seen in 25% of the cases, at 12 weeks in 90% and at 13–14 weeks in all cases[57]. The five-chamber, aortic arch and ductus arteriosus views were first seen in some fetuses from 12 weeks but, in the majority, only at 14 weeks. The aortic root in short-axis projection and the left ventricle in long-axis view could be imaged in 70% and 40% of fetuses, respectively by 12 weeks. Aortic and pulmonary valves were first visualized at 12 weeks in 20% of the cases[57]. Johnson et al. reported that the proportion of cases in which a full cardiac anatomic survey (four-chamber, aorta, pulmonary artery and pulmonary veins) was possible was 0% at 10–11 weeks, 31% at 12 weeks, 43% at 13 weeks and 46% at 14 weeks[59]. Gembruch et al. visualized the four-chamber view as well as the origin and double crossing of the aorta and pulmonary trunk in 67% of cases at 11 weeks, 80% at 12 weeks and 100% at 13–14 weeks[60].

There are several case reports on the sonographic diagnosis of cardiac defects at 11–14 weeks of gestation. Gembruch et al. reported an 11-week fetus with persistent bradycardia (60 bpm), increased nuchal translucency, complete atrioventricular canal defect and complete heart block; the pregnancy was terminated and pathological examination demonstrated situs inversus visceralis totalis and confirmed the septal defect[61]. DeVore et al. examined a 14-week fetus with persistent bradycardia (70 bpm) and found ventricular septal defect, ventricular wall hypertrophy, dilated aortic root, pericardial effusion, ascites and situs inversus of the stomach; pathological examination after intrauterine death at 16 weeks confirmed the ultrasound findings[62]. Bronshtein et al. reported the ultrasound findings in a 13-week fetus with ventricular septal defect and overriding aorta, suggesting the diagnosis of tetralogy of Fallot[63]. In addition, there was increased nuchal translucency thickness and exomphalos, and cytogenetic analysis demonstrated trisomy 18. Pathological examination after intrauterine death at 17 weeks confirmed the diagnosis of tetralogy of Fallot. In another case of exomphalos at 13 weeks, pericardial effusion and ventricular septal defect were identified; the fetal karyotype was normal. At 18 weeks, hydrocephalus and oligohydramnios were also noted and pathological examination after intrauterine death at 21 weeks confirmed the ultrasound findings and in addition, there was a double-outlet right ventricle and absence of the ductus arteriosus[63].

Achiron et al. reported the sonographic findings in eight fetuses with cardiac defects diagnosed at 10–12 weeks of gestation[64]. In seven of the cases, there was increased nuchal translucency thickness and pericardial effusion; the fetal karyotype was normal in seven and one had Turner syndrome. There was one case of tachycardia, one of ectopia cordis in association with exomphalos, one with a giant right atrium that, in subsequent pathological examination after termination of pregnancy, was diagnosed as Uhl disease, two cases with atrioventricular septal defects and three cases with ventricular septal defects; pathological examination in the latter group showed tetralogy of Fallot in two and persistent truncus arteriosus in the third[64].

Bronshtein et al. reported the results of an ultrasound screening study involving 81 fetuses at 12 weeks, 341 at 13 weeks and 980 at 14 weeks[65]. Five fetuses with cardiac defects were identified, including one with a small left ventricle and pericardial effusion at 11 weeks, one with ventricular septal defect, dilated left ventricle and pericardial effusion at 12 weeks that was subsequently diagnosed as tetralogy of Fallot, one with ventricular septal defect and overriding aorta at 13 weeks, one with dextrocardia at 14 weeks that was subsequently found to also have a ventricular septal defect, and another with a single atrium and single ventricle at 14 weeks.

Gembruch et al. reported the results of ultrasound screening in 15 fetuses at 11 weeks, 30 at 12 weeks, 51 at 13 weeks and 11 at 14 weeks[60]. There were ten fetuses with cardiac anomalies and, in nine of these, the diagnosis was correctly made at the 11–14-week scan; in one case, complete atrioventricular septal defect with double-outlet right ventricle was not detected at 12 weeks but was correctly diagnosed at 21 weeks. The defects identified were: five cases with complete atrioventricular septal defect, including one with dextrocardia and two with atrioventricular heart block; there was one case of single ventricle and common atrium that was subsequently, at the 20-week scan, also found to have dextrocardia, malposition of the great arteries and situs inversus visceralis; one case of perimembranous ventricular septal defect; one case with suspected single ventricle and hypoplasia of the aorta that was subsequently found at postmortem examination to have hypoplastic left heart, hypoplasia of the ascending aorta and the aortic arch, right-sided isomerism of the atria and asplenia; one case of hypoplastic left heart, hypoplastic aorta and left ventricular endocardial fibroelastosis. In eight of the ten cases with cardiac defects, there was increased nuchal translucency thickness; the fetal karyotype was normal in six cases, trisomy 21 in two, trisomy 18 in one and Turner syndrome in one[60].

Screening studies – relation to nuchal translucency thickness

In a study of 29 154 chromosomally normal, singleton pregnancies, 56% of major abnormalities of the heart and great arteries were found in the subgroup with nuchal translucency above the 95th centile[66]. Therefore, measurement of nuchal translucency thickness at 11–14 weeks may constitute the most effective method of screening for cardiac defects.

In patients with increased nuchal translucency, it is now possible to undertake detailed cardiac scanning in early pregnancy. A specialist scan from 14 weeks can effectively reassure the majority of parents that there is no major cardiac defect. In the cases with a major defect, the early scan can either lead to the correct diagnosis or at least raise suspicions so that follow-up scans are carried out. The scans can be performed either transvaginally or transabdominally. However, more important than the actual route for such a scan is the need to use high-quality equipment and, in particular, with facilities for color Doppler examination. At 14 weeks, the gray scale alone is not sufficient for accurate examination of the heart and it is necessary also to use color Doppler to confirm normal forward flow to both ventricles and to identify the outflow tracts.

ABDOMINAL WALL DEFECTS

Sonographically, the stomach is identified as a sonolucent cystic structure in the upper left quadrant of the abdomen. It is first visualized at 8–9 weeks and it is seen in all cases by 12–13 weeks[11,18,49]. At 8–10 weeks, of gestation, all fetuses demonstrate herniation of the midgut that is visualized as a hyperechogenic mass in the base of the umbilical cord; retraction into the abdominal cavity occurs at 10–12 weeks and it is completed by 11 weeks and 5 days[11,67,68].

Exomphalos

This is a sporadic abnormality with a birth prevalence of about 1 in 4000. Prenatal diagnosis by ultrasound is based on the demonstration of the mid-line anterior abdominal wall defect, the herniated sac with its visceral contents and the umbilical cord insertion

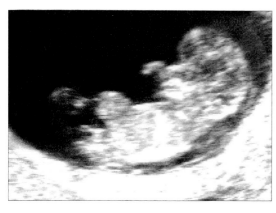

Figure 12 Exomphalos in a 12-week fetus

at the apex of the sac (Figure 12). Occasionally, there is an associated failure in the cephalic embryonic fold, resulting in the pentalogy of Cantrell (omphalocele, anterior diaphragmatic hernia, sternal cleft, ectopia cordis and cardiac defects) or failure of the caudal fold, in which case the omphalocele may be associated with exstrophy of the bladder or cloaca, imperforate anus, colonic atresia and sacral vertebral defects. Fetal exomphalos is associated with chromosomal defects, usually trisomy 18, in about 30% of cases at mid-gestation and in 15% of neonates.

Schmidt and Kubli described a case of exomphalos at 13 weeks as an echogenic tumor at the umbilicus; the fetus was subsequently found to have trisomy 18[19]. Brown et al. reported the diagnosis of exomphalos containing liver at 10 weeks, but retrospective examinations of the sonograms obtained at 6–9 weeks did not reveal any abnormality; the diagnosis was confirmed after delivery[69]. Similarly, Pagliano et al. reported the diagnosis of exomphalos containing liver and bowel in a 10-week fetus; the pregnancy was terminated and the diagnosis was confirmed[70]. Heydanus et al. reported the diagnosis of exomphalos in three fetuses at 12–14 weeks; in one there was an associated ectopia cordis and hydrops and the pregnancy was terminated, in the second there was an associated two-vessel cord and intrauterine death occurred and, in the third with isolated exomphalos, there was an infant death[71].

van Zalen-Sprock et al. reported the findings of 14 cases with exomphalos diagnosed at 11–14 weeks of gestation[68]. In eight cases, there was increased nuchal translucency thickness (3.5–10 mm) and seven of these had chromosomal abnormalities, mainly trisomy 18. The contents of the exomphalos were bowel only in the chromosomally abnormal group and liver as well as bowel in those with a normal karyotype. In the chromosomally normal group, there were four with other defects, such as tetralogy of Fallot and Meckel–Gruber syndrome; only three infants were liveborn.

Screening studies

An ultrasound screening study of 622 high-risk pregnancies at 10–13 weeks correctly diagnosed the two cases of exomphalos[25]. In two other screening studies of low-risk patients, involving 1632 pregnancies at 12–14 weeks[35] and 1473 pregnancies at 10–14 weeks[27], respectively, there were four cases of exomphalos (two in each) and they were all diagnosed in the first-trimester scan.

In a screening study for chromosomal abnormalities by assessment of fetal nuchal translucency thickness at 10–14 weeks of gestation, there were 15 726 pregnancies with a minimum gestation of 11 weeks and 4 days and, in this group, there were 18 cases of exomphalos[72]. In seven cases, the karyotype was normal, in nine there was trisomy 18, in one trisomy 13 and in one triploidy. Furthermore, in the total group, the prevalence of exomphalos in fetuses with trisomy 18 was 23%, in those with trisomy 13 it was 9%, in those with triploidy it was 13% and in those with no evidence of these chromosomal defects it was 0.045%. This study demonstrated that both the prevalence of exomphalos and the associated risk for chromosomal defects increase with maternal age and decrease with gestational age[72].

Gastroschisis

This is a sporadic defect with a birth prevalence of about 1 in 4000. Evisceration of the intestine occurs through a small abdominal wall defect located just lateral and usually to the right of an intact umbilical cord. Prenatal diagnosis by ultrasound is based on the demonstration of the normally situated umbilicus and the herniated loops of intestine, which are free-floating. Associated chromosomal abnormalities are rare.

Surprisingly, although the incidence of gastroschisis in ultrasound studies during the second trimester of pregnancy is similar to that of exomphalos, there is a sparsity of reports on first-trimester diagnosis. Kushnir *et al.* reported a 13-week fetus with a free-floating cauliflower-shaped mass protruding through the fetal abdomen and to the right of a normally inserted umbilical cord; the diagnosis was confirmed after delivery at term[73]. Similarly, Guzman reported a 12-week fetus with gastroschisis; there was spontaneous rupture of membranes and intrauterine death at 22 weeks[74].

Screening study

In an ultrasound screening study of 622 high-risk pregnancies at 10–13 weeks, there was one 11-week fetus with gastroschisis, encephalocele and kyphoscoliosis; the pregnancy was terminated[25].

URINARY TRACT DEFECTS

The fetal kidneys and adrenals can first be visualized by transabdominal ultrasound at 9 weeks and they are seen in all cases from 12 weeks[18]. The renal echogenicity is high at 9 weeks but decreases with gestation; the adrenals appear as translucent structures with an echodense cortex[18]. The fetal bladder can be visualized in about 80% of fetuses at 11 weeks and in more than 90% by 13 weeks[75]. At 12–13 weeks, the fetal kidneys can be visualized in 99% of the cases, by using both transabdominal and transvaginal sonography[49].

Bilateral renal agenesis

This sporadic condition, with a birth prevalence of about 1 in 4000, is usually diagnosed in the second trimester of pregnancy by the findings of anhydramnios, absence of the urinary bladder and failure to identify the fetal kidneys; the differential diagnosis is preterm prelabor rupture of membranes and severe uteroplacental insufficiency that may also present with oligohydramnios.

Bronshtein *et al.* reported the prenatal diagnosis of bilateral renal agenesis at 14 weeks of gestation in five fetuses; in all cases, there were hypoechogenic masses in the renal beds, that were subsequently found at pathological examination to be enlarged adrenals[76]. The amniotic fluid volume was normal in all cases at 14 weeks. In two cases, a cystic structure suggestive of the fetal bladder was temporarily detected in the fetal pelvis but this disappeared by 16–17 weeks.

Infantile polycystic kidney disease

This an autosomal recessive condition with a birth prevalence of about 1 in 50 000. It is subdivided into perinatal, neonatal, infantile and juvenile types, on the basis of the age of onset of the clinical presentation and the degree of renal involvement. Prenatal diagnosis by ultrasound is confined to the perinatal and probably the neonatal types and is based on the demonstration of bilaterally enlarged and homogeneously hyper-echogenic kidneys. While there is often associated oligohydramnios, this is not found invariably. These sonographic appearances, however, may not become apparent until 26 weeks of gestation, and therefore serial scans should be performed for exclusion of the diagnosis.

Bronshtein *et al.* reported a case of infantile polycystic kidney disease; at 11 and 15 weeks, the kidneys and bladder looked normal, but at 28 weeks there was oligohydramnios with bilaterally enlarged and diffusely hyperechogenic kidneys[77].

Retrospective examination of the videotapes taken from the early scans demonstrated that the kidneys were of increased echogenicity and increased length from as early as 12 weeks.

Multicystic dysplastic kidney disease

In this sporadic condition, which may be unilateral or bilateral, the collecting tubules and nephrons are dysplastic. The collecting tubules become cystic and the diameter of the cysts determines the size of the kidneys, which may be large and multicystic or small, shrunken and hyperechogenic. Occasionally, only one of a small number of adjacent collecting tubules is involved so that only a segment of the kidney is abnormal. With bilateral involvement, there is associated absence of the bladder and oligohydramnios.

Cullen *et al.* reported a case that at 11 weeks demonstrated hyperechoic kidneys with no obvious dilatation of the bladder; ultrasound examination in the newborn, after delivery at term, confirmed the diagnosis of cystic dysplastic kidneys[25]. Bronshtein *et al.* reported a case with a unilateral multicystic kidney diagnosed at 12 weeks during routine ultrasound examination; the fetal karyotype was normal[78]. Ultrasound examination of the newborn confirmed the antenatal diagnosis.

Screening studies

In a screening study involving ultrasound examinations at 11–14 weeks of gestation and at 18–20 weeks in 3991 patients, there were three cases of unilateral multicystic dysplastic kidneys and none was detected at the early scan; two were diagnosed at 18–20 weeks and the third was detected at 31 weeks[26]. In another screening study involving 1632 pregnancies at 12–14 weeks, there was one case with unilateral multicystic kidneys and this was correctly identified in the first-trimester scan[35].

Hydronephrosis

Varying degrees of pelvicalyceal dilatation are found in about 1% of fetuses. Mild hydronephrosis or pyelectasia may be due to relaxation of smooth muscle of the urinary tract by the high levels of circulating maternal hormones, or maternal–fetal overhydration. In the majority of cases, the condition remains stable or resolves in the neonatal period. In about 20% of cases, there may be an underlying ureteropelvic junction obstruction or vesicoureteric reflux that requires postnatal follow-up and possible surgery. Moderate or severe pelvicalyceal dilatation is usually progressive and, in more than 50% of cases, surgery is necessary during the first 2 years of life.

Screening studies

In an ultrasound screening study of 622 high-risk pregnancies at 10–13 weeks, there were two cases of hydronephrosis and exomphalos and they were both detected at the first scan; one pregnancy was terminated and the other resulted in a livebirth with cloacal defect as well as the exomphalos[25]. In a screening study involving ultrasound examinations at 11–14 weeks of gestation and at 18–20 weeks in 3991 low-risk patients, there were four cases of hydronephrosis and only one of these was diagnosed at the early scan[26].

Megacystis

Sebire *et al.* examined transabdominally 300 pregnancies at 10–14 weeks of gestation and reported a significant increase in bladder length with crown–rump length (Figure 13), but, within this gestational age range, none of the measurements was more than 6 mm[79]. The fetal bladder was always visualized if the crown–rump length was more than 67 mm, but not in 9% of those with a crown–rump length of 38–67 mm.

Bulic *et al.* described a 14-week fetus with megacystis (bladder length 50 mm) and oligohydramnios; pathological examination after termination at 15 weeks showed urethral atresia, hypertrophic bladder, dysplastic kidneys and absence of abdominal musculature[80]. In another 11-week fetus, there was megacystis (20 mm); at 14 weeks there was enlargement of the bladder and oligohydramnios. Pathological examination after termination demonstrated urethral atresia, severe megacystis but normal kidneys[80].

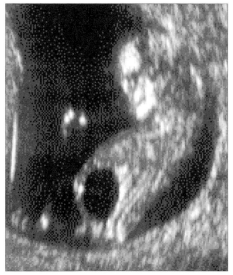

Figure 13 Megacystis in a 12-week fetus

Stiller reported an 11-week fetus with megacystis (10 mm) but normal kidneys and amniotic fluid[81]. At 13 weeks, there was enlargement of the bladder (30 mm) and bilateral hydronephrosis with reduced amniotic fluid; the pregnancy was terminated.

Drugan *et al.* reported a 12-week fetus with megacystis (18 mm); at 14 weeks there was further enlargement of the bladder with normal kidneys but oligohydramnios[82]. Vesicoamniotic shunting was carried out and the pregnancy continued normally; a male infant with mild prune-belly and moderate renal function (40–50%) was born at 35 weeks.

Zimmer and Bronshtein reported an 11-week fetus with megacystis (13 mm) and two umbilical cord cysts[83]. At 12 weeks, the bladder increased (30 mm) and there was evidence of hydronephrosis; at 13 weeks there was intrauterine death. In another 12-week fetus, there was megacystis (46 mm), bilateral hydronephrosis, increased nuchal translucency and talipes. Chorionic villus sampling showed Turner mosaicism and the pregnancy was terminated.

Yoshida *et al.* reported a 13-week fetus with megacystis (45 mm) and decreased amniotic fluid volume; follow-up scans demonstrated resolution of the megacystis and normalization of the amniotic fluid volume[84]. At 28 weeks, tetralogy of Fallot was diagnosed. Investigations after delivery at 38 weeks confirmed the cardiac defect and, in addition, demonstrated vaginal atresia, imperforate anus, recto-urethral fistula, bilateral vesicoureteral reflux, unilateral renal hypoplasia, hypoplasia of abdominal muscles, scoliosis and bilateral talipes. The karyotype was normal female. The suggested diagnosis was VACTERL-like association.

Fried *et al.* reported a 13-week fetus with megacystis (30 mm); a repeat scan 2 days later demonstrated urinary ascites with a thick-walled deflated bladder and the pregnancy was terminated[85]. The fetal karyotype was 46,XY.

Hoshino *et al.* reported a fetus with normal sonographic appearance at 10 weeks but, at 12 weeks, there was megacystis (40 mm) with normal amniotic fluid volume; at 13 weeks, the diameter of the bladder increased to 54 mm, there was bilateral hydronephrosis and the amniotic fluid volume was reduced[86].

Cazorla *et al.* reported a fetus with normal sonographic appearance at 8 weeks but, at 13 weeks, there was megacystis (33 mm) and reduced amniotic fluid volume; the fetal karyotype was 46,XY[87]. At 16 weeks, the fetus developed generalized edema and the pregnancy was terminated. Pathological examination revealed urethral atresia, megacystis, hydronephrosis and atrophied abdominal muscles.

Screening studies

In an ultrasound screening study of 622 high-risk pregnancies at 10–13 weeks, there were two cases with urethral obstruction presenting as megacystis at 11 and 13 weeks of gestation[25]. In a screening study for chromosomal abnormalities by assessment of fetal nuchal translucency thickness, 24 492 singleton pregnancies were examined[79]. Megacystis was present in 15 fetuses (prevalence of 1 in 1633) and, in these cases, the longitudinal bladder diameter was 8–32 mm. There were three cases with chromosomal abnormalities and two of these had increased nuchal translucency thickness. In the chromosomally normal group with mild-to-moderate megacystis (longitudinal bladder diameter of 8–12 mm), the majority of fetuses had spontaneous resolution without any obvious adverse effects on renal development and function. In those with severe megacystis (minimum longitudinal bladder diameter of 17 mm), there was evolution to obstructive uropathy and renal dysplasia[79].

Extensive animal studies have demonstrated that obstructive uropathy causes renal dysplasia and the degree of renal damage is related both to the onset and duration of the obstruction[88,89]. Furthermore, such studies have shown that renal damage can be reduced by intrauterine surgery to by-pass the obstruction. However, the data from vesico–amniotic shunting in human fetuses with obstructive uropathy have not provided conclusive evidence that such interventions are beneficial, possibly because, by mid-gestation, when surgery is usually undertaken, irreversible renal damage may have already occurred. The extent to which first-trimester diagnosis of megacystis and vesico–amniotic shunting could prevent the subsequent development of renal damage remains to be determined.

SKELETAL DEFECTS

Limb buds are first seen by ultrasound at about the 8th week of gestation, the femur and humerus are seen from 9 weeks, tibia/fibula and radius/ulna from 10 weeks and digits of hands and feet from 11 weeks; all long bones are consistently seen from 11 weeks[14,18,90,91]. Body movements (wiggling) are seen at 9 weeks and, by 11 weeks, limbs move about readily[18,90]. The length of the humerus, radius/ulna, femur and tibia/fibula are similar at 11–14 weeks and increase linearly with gestation from about 6 mm at 11 weeks to 13 mm at 14 weeks; the femur to foot ratio is 0.85[92].

Skeletal dysplasias are found in about 1 per 4000 births; about 25% of affected fetuses are stillborn and about 30% die in the neonatal period. The most common dysplasias are thanatophoric dysplasia, osteogenesis imperfecta, achondroplasia, achondrogenesis and asphyxiating thoracic dysplasia. Several case reports have described the prenatal diagnosis of a wide range of skeletal defects in the first trimester of pregnancy and they are usually associated with increased nuchal translucency thickness (see Chapter 2).

Caudal regression syndrome

This rare, sporadic syndrome presents with varying degrees of vertebral anomalies from partial sacral agenesis to complete absence of the lumbosacral spine. Sirenomelia is the extreme form, with variable fusion and hypoplasia of the lower extremities and genito-urinary, gastrointestinal, cardiovascular and central nervous system abnormalities. It is 250 times more common in poorly controlled diabetic mothers than in the general population.

Baxi *et al.* performed serial ultrasound scans in a patient that originally presented in diabetic ketoacidotic coma[93]. At 9 weeks, the crown–rump length was shorter by a week than expected from the menstrual age. At 11 weeks, there was a protuberence of the lower spine and no normal movements of the thighs were seen. At 14 weeks, the femora were fixed in a 'frog-leg' position and were never seen moving independently from each other. At 17 weeks, shortening and kyphosis of the lower spine were observed. Pathological examination after termination of the pregnancy confirmed the diagnosis of caudal regression syndrome.

REFERENCES

1. Moore GW, Hutchins GM, O'Rahilly R. The estimated age of staged human embryos and early fetuses. *Am J Obstet Gynecol* 1981;139:500–6
2. O'Rahilly R, Müller F. *Developmental Stages in Human Embryos.* Washington DC: Carnegie Institute Publ, 1987
3. Timor-Tritsch IE, Peisner DB, Raju S. Sonoembryology: an organ-oriented approach using a high-frequency vaginal probe. *J Clin Ultrasound* 1990;18:286–98
4. O'Rahilly R, Müller F. *The Embryonic Human Brain. An Atlas of Developmental Stages.* New York: Wiley-Liss, 1994
5. Blumenfeld Z, Rottem S, Elgali S, Timor-Tritsch IE. Transvaginal sonographic assessment of early embryological development. In Timor-Tritsch IE, Rottem S, eds. *Transvaginal Sonography,* London: Heinemann Medical Books, 1988:87–108
6. Bree RL, Marn CS. Transvaginal sonography in the first trimester: embryology, anatomy, and hCG correlation. *Sem Ultrasound, CT, MR* 1990;11:12–21
7. Blaas HG, Eik-Nes SH, Kiserud T, Hellevik LR. Early development of the forebrain and midbrain: a longitudinal ultrasound study from 7 to 12 weeks of gestation. *Ultrasound Obstet Gynecol* 1994;4: 183–92
8. Wisser J, Dirschedl P. Embryonic heart rate in dated human embryos. *Early Hum Dev* 1994;37: 107–15

9. Wisser J, Dirschedl P, Krone S. Estimation of gestational age by transvaginal sonographic measurements of greatest embryonic length in dated human embryos. *Ultrasound Obstet Gynecol* 1994;4: 457–62

10. Blaas HG, Eik-Nes SH, Kiserud T, Hellevik LR. Early development of the hindbrain: a longitudinal ultrasound study from 7 to 12 weeks of gestation. *Ultrasound Obstet Gynecol* 1995;5:151–60

11. Blaas HG, Eik-Nes SH, Kiserud T, Hellevik LR. Early development of the hindbrain: a longitudinal ultrasound study from 7 to 12 weeks of gestation. *Ultrasound Obstet Gynecol* 1995;6:240–9

12. Blaas HG, Eik-Nes SH, Berg S, Torp H. In-vivo three-dimensional ultrasound reconstructions of embryos and early fetuses. *Lancet* 1998;352:1182–6

13. Blaas HG, Eik-Nes SH, Bremnes JB. Embryonic growth. A longitudinal biometric ultrasound study. *Ultrasound Obstet Gynecol* 1998;12:346–54

14. van Zalen-Sprock RM, van Brons JTJ, van Vugt JMG, van Harten HJ, van Gijn HP. Ultrasonographic and radiologic visualization of the developing embryonic skeleton. *Ultrasound Obstet Gynecol* 1997;9:392–7

15. Campbell S, Holt EM, Johnson FD. Anencephaly: early ultrasonic diagnosis and active management. *Lancet* 1972;2:1226–7

16. Warkany J. Anencephaly. In Warkany J, ed. *Congenital Malformations*. Chicago: Yearbook Publishers, 1971:189–200

17. O' Rahilly R, Gardner E. The initial appearance of ossification in staged human embryos. *Am J Anat* 1974;134:291–308

18. Green JJ, Hobbins JC. Abdominal ultrasound examination of the first trimester fetus. *Am J Obstet Gynecol* 1988;159:165–75

19. Schmidt W, Kubli F. Early diagnosis of severe congenital malformations by ultrasonography. *J Perinat Med* 1982;10:233–41

20. Johnson A, Losure TA, Weiner S. Early diagnosis of anencephaly. *J Clin Ultrasound* 1985;13:503–5

21. Rottem S, Bronshtein M, Thaler I, Brandes JM. First trimester transvaginal sonographic diagnosis of fetal anomalies. *Lancet* 1989;1:444–5

22. Kennedy KA, Flick KJ, Thurmond AS. First-trimester diagnosis of exencephaly. *Am J Obstet Gynecol* 1990;162:461–3

23. Bronshtein M, Ornoy A. Acrania: anencephaly resulting from secondary degeneration of a closed neural tube: two cases in the same family. *J Clin Ultrasound* 1991;19:230–4

24. Goldstein RB, Filly RA, Callen PW. Sonography of anencephaly: pitfalls in early diagnosis. *J Clin Ultrasound* 1989;17:397–402

25. Cullen MT, Green J, Whetham J, Salafia C, Gabrielli S, Hobbins JC. Transvaginal ultrasonographic detection of congenital anomalies in the first trimester. *Am J Obstet Gynecol* 1990;163:466–76

26. Hernadi L, Torocsik M. Screening for fetal anomalies in the 12th week of pregnancy by transvaginal sonography in an unselected population. *Prenat Diagn* 1997;17:753–9

27. Pajkrt E, van Lith JMM, Mol BWJ, Bleker OP, Bilardo CM. Screening for Down's syndrome by fetal nuchal translucency measurement in a general obstetric population. *Ultrasound Obstet Gynecol* 1998;12:163–9

28. Chatzipapas IK, Whitlow BJ, Economides DL. The 'Mickey Mouse' sign and the diagnosis of anencephaly in early pregnancy. *Ultrasound Obstet Gynecol* 1998;13:196–9

29. Johnson SP, Sebire NJ, Snijders RJM, Tunkel S, Nicolaides KH. Ultrasound screening for anencephaly at 10–14 weeks of gestation. *Ultrasound Obstet Gynecol* 1197;9:14–16

30. van Zalen-Sprock RM, van Vugt JMG, van Geijn HP. First-trimester sonographic detection of neurodevelopmental abnormalities in some single-gene disorders. *Prenat Diagn* 1996;16:199–202

31. Bronshtein M, Zimmer EZ. Transvaginal sonographic follow-up on the formation of fetal cephalocele at 13–19 weeks' gestation. *Obstet Gynecol* 1991;78:528–30

32. van Zalen-Sprock M, van Vugt JMG, van der Harten HJ, van Geijn HP. Cephalocele and cystic hygroma: diagnosis and differentiation in the first trimester of pregnancy with transvaginal sonography. Report of two cases. *Ultrasound Obstet Gynecol* 1992;2:289–92

33. Pachi A, Giancotti A, Torcia F, de Prosperi V, Maggi E. Meckel–Gruber syndrome: ultrasonographic diagnosis at 13 weeks' gestational age in an at-risk case. *Prenat Diagn* 1989;9:187–90

34. Sepulveda W, Sebire NJ, Souka A, Snijders RJM, Nicolaides KH. Diagnosis of the Meckel–Gruber syndrome at eleven to fourteen weeks' gestation. *Am J Obstet Gynecol* 1997;176:316–19

35. Economides DL, Braithwaite JM. First trimester ultrasonographic diagnosis of fetal structural abnormalities in a low risk population. *Br J Obstet Gynaecol* 1998;105:53–7

36. Braithwaite J, Economides DL. First-trimester diagnosis of Meckel–Gruber syndrome by transabdominal sonography in a low-risk case. *Prenat Diagn* 1995;15:1168–70

37. Timor-Tritsch IE, Monteagudo A, Warren WB. Transvaginal sonographic definition of the central nervous system in the first and early second trimesters. *Am J Obstet Gynecol* 1991;164:497–503

38. Kushnir U, Shalev J, Bronshtein M, Bider D, Lipitz S, Nebel L, Mashiach S, Ben-Rafael Z. Fetal intracranial anatomy in the first trimester of pregnancy: transvaginal ultrasonographic evaluation. *Neuroradiology* 1989;31:222–5

39. Ulm B, Ulm MR, Deutinger J, Bernaschek G. Dandy–Walker malformation diagnosed before 21 weeks of gestation: associated malformations and chromosomal abnormalities. *Ultrasound Obstet Gynecol* 1997;10:167–70

40. Lin Y, Chang F, Liu C. Antenatal detection of hydranencephaly at 12 weeks, menstrual age. *J Clin Ultrasound* 1992;20:62–4

41. Toth Z, Csecsei K, Szeifert G, Torok O, Papp Z. Early prenatal diagnosis of cyclopia associated with holoprosencephaly. *J Clin Ultrasound* 1986;14:550–3

42. Bronshtein M, Wiener Z. Early transvaginal sonographic diagnosis of alobar holoprosencephaly. *Prenat Diagn* 1991;11:459–62

43. Gonzalez-Gomez F, Salamanca A, Padilla MC, Camara M, Sabatel RM. Alobar holoprosencephalic embryo detected via transvaginal sonography. *Eur J Obstet Gynecol Reprod Biol* 1992;47:266–70

44. Sakala EP, Gaio KL. Fundal uterine leiomyoma obscuring first trimester transabdominal sonographic diagnosis of fetal holoprosencephaly. *J Reprod Med* 1993;38:400–2

45. Turner CD, Silva S, Jeanty P. Prenatal diagnosis of alobar holoprosencephaly at 10 weeks of gestation. *Ultrasound Obstet Gynecol* 1999;13:360–2

46. Wong HS, Lam YH, Tang MHY, Cheung LWK, Ng LKL, Yan KW. First-trimester ultrasound diagnosis of holoprosencephaly: three case reports. *Ultrasound Obstet Gynecol* 1999;13:356–9

47. Snijders RJM, Sebire NJ, Nayar R, Souka A, Nicolaides KH. Increased nuchal translucency in trisomy 13 fetuses at 10–14 weeks of gestation. *Am J Med Genet* 1999;in press

48. Sherer DM, Hearn-Stebbins B, Harvey W, Metlay LA, Abramowicz JS. Endovaginal sonographic diagnosis of iniencephaly apertus and craniorachischisis at 13 weeks, menstrual age. *J Clin Ultrasound* 1993;21:124–7

49. Braithwaite JM, Armstrong MA, Economides DL. Assessment of fetal anatomy at 12 to 13 weeks of gestation by transabdominal and transvaginal sonography. *Br J Obstet Gynaecol* 1996;103:82–5

50. Campbell S, Pryse-Davies J, Coltard TM, *et al.* Ultrasound in the diagnosis of spina bifida. *Lancet* 1975;1:1065–6

51. Roberts CJ, Evans KT, Hibbard BM, Laurence KM, Roberts EE, Robertson IB. Diagnostic effectiveness of ultrasound in detection of neural tube defect: the South Wales experience of 2509 scans (1977–1982) in high-risk mothers. *Lancet* 1983;ii:1068–9

52. Nicolaides KH, Campbell S, Gabbe SG, Guidetti R. Ultrasound screening for spina bifida: cranial and cerebellar signs. *Lancet* 1986;2:72–4

53. Blumenfeld Z, Siegler E, Bronshtein M. The early diagnosis of neural tube defects. *Prenat Diagn* 1993;13:863–71

54. Sebire NJ, Noble PL, Thorpe-Beeston JG, Snijders RJM, Nicolaides KH. Presence of the 'lemon sign' in fetuses with spina bifida at the 10–14-week scan. *Ultrasound Obstet Gynecol* 1997;10:403–5

55. Bernard JP, Suarez B, Rambaud C, Muller F, Ville Y. Prenatal diagnosis of neural tube defect before 12 weeks' gestation: direct and indirect ultrasonographic semeiology. *Ultrasound Obstet Gynecol* 1997;10:406–9

56. Tegnander E, Eik-Nes SH, Johansen OJ, Linker DT. Prenatal detection of heart defects at the routine fetal examination at 18 weeks in a non-selected poulation. *Ultrasound Obstet Gynecol* 1995; 5:372–80

57. Dolkart LA, Reimers FT. Transvaginal fetal echocardiography in early pregnancy: normative data. *Am J Obstet Gynecol* 1991;165:688–91

58. Bronshtein M, Siegler E, Eshcoli Z, Zimmer EZ. Transvaginal ultrasound measurements of the fetal heart at 11 to 17 weeks of gestation. *Am J Perinat* 1992;9:38–42

59. Johnson P, Sharland G, Maxwell D, Allan L. The role of transvaginal sonography in the early detection of congenital heart disease. *Ultrasound Obstet Gynecol* 1992;2:248–51

60. Gembruch U, Knopfle G, Bald R, Hansmann M. Early diagnosis of fetal congenital heart disease by transvaginal echocardiography. *Ultrasound Obstet Gynecol* 1993;3:310–17

61. Gembruch U, Knopfle G, Chatterjee M, Bald R, Hansmann M. First-trimester diagnosis of fetal congenital heart disease by transvaginal two-dimensional and Doppler echocardiography. *Obstet Gynecol* 1990;75:496–8

62. DeVore GR, Steiger GR, Larson EJ. Fetal echocardiography: the prenatal diagnosis of a ventricular septal defect in a 14-week fetus with pulmonary artery hypoplasia. *Obstet Gynecol* 1987;69:494–7

63. Bronshtein M, Siegler E, Yoffe N, Zimmer EZ. Prenatal diagnosis of ventricular septal defect and overriding aorta at 14 weeks' gestation, using transvaginal sonography. *Prenat Diagn* 1990;10:697–702

64. Achiron R, Rotstein Z, Lipitz S, Mashiach S, Hegesh J. First-trimester diagnosis of fetal congenital heart disease by transvaginal ultrasonography. *Obstet Gynecol* 1994;84:69–72

65. Bronshtein M, Zimmer EZ, Milo S, Ho SY, Lorber A, Gerlis M. Fetal cardiac abnormalities detected by transvaginal sonography at 12–16 weeks' gestation. *Obstet Gynecol* 1991;78:374–8

66. Hyett JA, Perdu M, Sharland GK, Snijders RJM, Nicolaides KH. Using fetal nuchal translucency to screen for major congenital cardiac defects at 10–14 weeks of gestation: population based cohort study. *Br Med J* 1999:318:81–5

67. Timor-Tritsch IE, Warren W, Peisner DB, Pirrone E. First-trimester midgut herniation: a high frequency transvaginal sonographic study. *Am J Obstet Gynecol* 1989;161:831–3

68. van Zalen-Sprock RM, van Vugt JMG, van Geijn HP. First-trimester sonography of physiological midgut herniation and early diagnosis of omphalocele. *Prenat Diagn* 1997;17:511–18

145

69. Brown DL, Emerson DS, Shulman LP, Carson SA. Sonographic diagnosis of omphalocele during the 10th week of gestation. *Am J Radiol* 1989;153:825–6

70. Pagliano M, Mossetti M, Ragno P. Echographic diagnosis of omphalocele in the first trimester of pregnancy. *J Clin Ultrasound* 1990;18:658–60

71. Heydanus R, Raats AM, Tibboel D, Lost FJ, Wladimiroff JW. Prenatal diagnosis of fetal abdominal wall defects: a retrospective analysis of 44 cases. *Prenat Diagn* 1996;16:411–17

72. Snijders RJM, Sebire NJ, Souka A, Santiago C, Nicolaides KH. Fetal exomphalos and chromosomal defects: relationship to maternal age and gestation. *Ultrasound Obstet Gynecol* 1995;6:250–5

73. Kushnir O, Izquierdo L, Vigil D, Curet LB. Early transvaginal diagnosis of gastroschisis. *J Clin Ultrasound* 1990;18:194–7

74. Guzman ER. Early prenatal diagnosis of gastroschisis with transvaginal sonography. *Am J Obstet Gynecol* 1990;162:1253–4

75. Rosati P, Guariglia L. Transvaginal sonographic assessment of the fetal urinary tract in early pregnancy. *Ultrasound Obstet Gynecol* 1996;7:95–100

76. Bronshtein M, Amit A, Achiron R, Noy I, Blumenfeld Z. The early prenatal sonographic diagnosis of renal agenesis: techniques and possible pitfalls. *Prenat Diagn* 1994;14:291–7

77. Bronshtein M, Bar-Hava I, Blumenfeld Z. Clues and pitfalls in the early prenatal diagnosis of 'late onset' infantile polycystic kidney. *Prenat Diagn* 1992;12:293–8

78. Bronshtein M, Yoffe N, Brandes JM, Blumenfeld Z. First and early second-trimester diagnosis of fetal urinary tract anomalies using transvaginal sonography. *Prenat Diagn* 1990;10:653–66

79. Sebire NJ, von Kaisenberg C, Rubio C, Snijders RJM, Nicolaides KH. Fetal megacystis at 10–14 weeks of gestation. *Ultrasound Obstet Gynecol* 1996;8: 387–90

80. Bulic M, Podobnik M, Korenic B, Bistricki J. First-trimester diagnosis of low obstructive uropathy: an indicator of initial renal function in the fetus. *J Clin Ultrasound* 1987;15:537–41

81. Stiller R. Early ultrasonic appearance of fetal bladder outlet obstruction. *Am J Obstet Gynecol* 1989;160:584–5

82. Drugan A, Zador IE, Bhatia RK, Sacks AJ, Evans M. First trimester diagnosis and early in utero treatment of obstructive uropathy. *Acta Obstet Gynecol Scand* 1989;68:645–9

83. Zimmer EZ, Bronshtein M. Fetal intra-abdominal cysts detected in the first and early second trimester by transvaginal sonography. *J Clin Ultrasound* 1991;19:564–7

84. Yoshida M, Matsumura M, Shintaku Y, Yura Y, Kanamori T, Matsushita K, Nonogaki T, Hayashi M, Tauchi K. Prenatally diagnosed female Prune-belly syndrome associated with tetralogy of Fallot. *Gynecol Obstet Invest* 1995;39:141–4

85. Fried S, Appelman Z, Caspi B. The origin of ascites in prune belly syndrome – early sonographic evidence. *Prenat Diagn* 1995;15:876–7

86. Hoshino T, Ihara Y, Shirane H, Ota T. Prenatal diagnosis of prune belly syndrome at 12 weeks of pregnancy: case report and review of the literature. *Ultrasound Obstet Gynecol* 1998;12:362–6

87. Cazorla E, Ruiz F, Abad A, Monleon J. Prune belly syndrome: early antenatal diagnosis. *Eur J Obstet Gynecol* 1997;72:31–3

88. Harrison MR, Nakayama DK, Noall R, De Lorimer AA. Correction of congenital hydronephrosis in utero. II. Decompression reverses the effect of obstruction on the fetal lung and urinary tract. *J Pediatr Surg* 1982;17:965–74

89. Glick PL, Harrison MR, Adzick NS, Noall RA, Villa RL. Correction of congenital hydronephrosis in utero. IV. In utero decompression prevents renal dysplasia. *J Pediatr Surg* 1984;19:649–57

90. Timor-Tritsch IE, Farine D, Rosen M. A close look at early embryonic development with the high-frequency transvaginal transducer. *Am J Obstet Gynecol* 1988;159:676–81

91. Timor-Tritsch IE, Monteagudo A, Peisner DB. High-frequency transvaginal sonographic examination for the potential malformation assessment of the 9-week to 14-week fetus. *J Clin Ultrasound* 1992;20:231–8

92. Zorzoli A, Kusterman E, Carvelli E, Corso FE, Fogliani R, Aimi G, Nicolini U. Measurements of fetal limb bones in early pregnancy. *Ultrasound Obstet Gynecol* 1994;4:29–33

93. Baxi L, Warren W, Collins M, Timor-Tritsch IE. Early detection of caudal regression syndrome with transvaginal scanning. *Obstet Gynecol* 1990;75:485–9

5

Multiple pregnancy

TYPES OF MULTIPLE PREGNANCY

Multiple pregnancy usually results from the ovulation and subsequent fertilization of more than one oocyte. In such cases, the fetuses are genetically different (polyzygotic or non-identical). Multiple pregnancy can also result from the splitting of one embryonic mass to form two or more genetically identical fetuses (monozygotic).

In all cases of polyzygotic multiple pregnancy, each zygote develops its own amnion, chorion and placenta (polychorionic). In monozygotic pregnancies, there may be sharing of the same placenta (monochorionic), amniotic sac (monoamniotic) or even fetal organs (conjoined or Siamese). When the single embryonic mass splits into two within 3 days of fertilization, which occurs in one-third of monozygotic twins, each fetus has its own amniotic sac and placenta (diamniotic and dichorionic) (Figure 1). When embryonic splitting occurs after the third day following fertilization, there are vascular communications within the two placental circulations (mono-chorionic). Embryonic splitting after the 9th day following fertilization results in monoamniotic, monochorionic twins and splitting after the 12th day results in conjoined twins.

INCIDENCE AND EPIDEMIOLOGY

Twins account for about 1% of all pregnancies, with two-thirds being dizygotic and one-third monozygotic. The incidence of dizygotic twins varies with ethnic group (up to 5 times higher in certain parts of Africa and half as high in parts of Asia), maternal age (2% at 35 years), parity (2% after four pregnancies) and method of conception (20% with ovulation induction). The incidence of monozygotic twins is similar in all ethnic groups and does not vary with maternal age or parity, but may be 2–3 times higher following *in vitro* fertilization procedures, possibly because with these methods the architecture of the zona pellucida is altered[1,2].

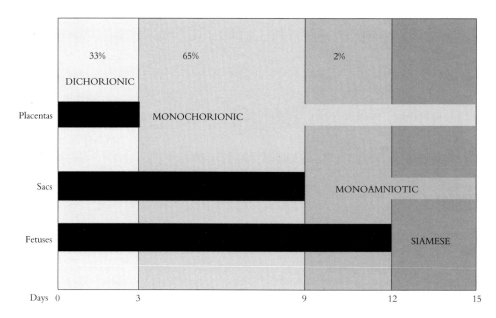

Figure 1 In monozygotic twins, embryonic splitting within the first 3 days after fertilization results in a diamniotic and dichorionic pregnancy; splitting between days 3 and 9 results in a diamniotic, monochorionic pregnancy; splitting between days 9 and 12 results in a mono-amniotic, monochorionic pregnancy; and splitting after the 12th day results in conjoined twins

In the last 20 years, the rate of twinning has increased (Figure 2). The increase in dizygotic twins is mainly due to the widespread use of assisted reproductive techniques and the increasing maternal age. There has also been an increase in the rate of mono-zygotic twinning, particularly in those countries in which there is widespread use of oral contraceptives.

The incidence of spontaneous multifetal (more than two) pregnancies can be derived from Hellin's rule (1 in 80^{n-1} pregnancies, where n is the number of fetuses). In recent years assisted reproductive techniques, such as ovulation induction and *in vitro* fertilization, have become important causes of multiple pregnancies and the vast majority of multifetal pregnancies result from such treatments.

ZYGOSITY AND CHORIONICITY

Zygosity can only be determined by DNA fingerprinting. Prenatally, such testing would require an invasive procedure to sample amniotic fluid (amniocentesis), placental tissue (chorionic villus sampling) or fetal blood (cordocentesis).

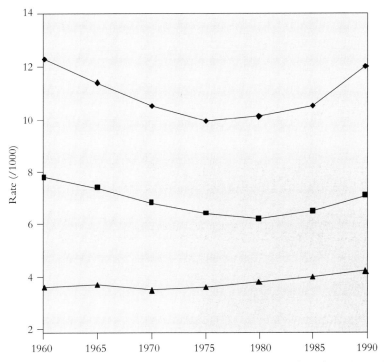

Figure 2 Twinning rate (per 1000 pregnancies) in England and Wales, 1960–1990 for all twins (diamond markers), dizygotic twins (square markers) and monozygotic twins (triangle markers); adapted from Derom *et al.*[3]

Determination of chorionicity can be performed by ultrasonography and relies on the assessment of fetal gender, number of placentas and characteristics of the membrane between the two amniotic sacs. Different-sex twins are dizygotic and therefore dichorionic, but in about two-thirds of twin pregnancies the fetuses are of the same sex and these may be either monozygotic or dizygotic. Similarly, if there are two separate placentas, the pregnancy is dichorionic, but, in the majority of cases, the two placentas are adjacent to each other and there are often difficulties in distinguishing between dichorionic-fused and monochorionic placentas.

In dichorionic twins, the intertwin membrane is composed of a central layer of chorionic tissue sandwiched between two layers of amnion, whereas in monochorionic twins there is no chorionic layer. Consequently, the intertwin membrane tends to be thicker and more echogenic in dichorionic than monochorionic pregnancies, but this is a subjective and quite unreliable finding. For example, one study reported that dichorionicity is associated with an inter-twin septum thickness of 2 mm or more[4], but the reproducibility of this measurement was poor and is dependent on such technical aspects as the angle of insonation and gestational age[5].

The best way to determine chorionicity is by an ultrasound examination at 6–9 weeks of gestation, when in dichorionic twins there is a thick septum between the chorionic sacs (Figure 3)[6–8]. After 9 weeks, this septum becomes progressively thinner to form the chorionic component of the intertwin membrane, but it remains thick and easy to identify at the base of the membrane as a triangular tissue projection, or lambda sign[9–11].

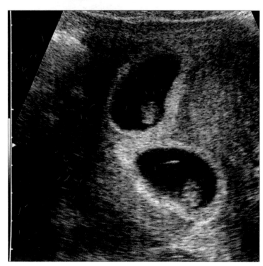

Figure 3 Dichorionic twin pregnancy at 8 weeks, demonstrating the thick septum

At 11–14 weeks of gestation, sonographic examination of the base of the inter-twin membrane for the presence or absence of the lambda sign (Figure 4) provides reliable distinction between dichorionic and monochorionic pregnancies. In an ultrasound study of 368 twin pregnancies at 10–14 weeks of gestation, pregnancies were classified as monochorionic if there was a single placental mass in the absence of the lambda sign at the inter-twin membrane–placental junction, and dichorionic if there was a single placental mass but the lambda sign was present or the placentas were not adjacent to each other[11]. In 81 (22%) cases, the pregnancies were classified as monochorionic and in 287 (78%) as dichorionic. All pregnancies classified as monochorionic resulted in the delivery of same-sex twins and all different-sex pairs were correctly classified as dichorionic[11].

Evolution of the lambda sign with gestation

With advancing gestation, there is regression of the chorion laeve and the lambda sign becomes progressively more difficult to identify. A study examined 154 twin pregnancies for the presence or absence of the lambda sign at 10–14 weeks of gestation

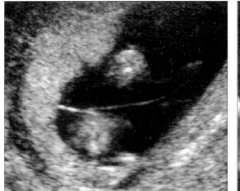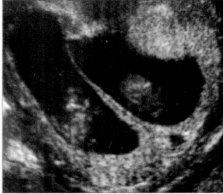

Figure 4 Ultrasound appearance of monochorionic (left) and dichorionic (right) twin pregnancies at 12 weeks of gestation. Note that, in both types, there appears to be a single placental mass but in the dichorionic type there is an extention of placental tissue into the base of the intertwin membrane, forming the lambda sign

and again at 16 and 20 weeks[12]. There were 101 twin pregnancies with a lambda sign identified at 10–14 weeks; at 16 weeks, the lambda sign was present in 98% of the cases and at 20 weeks in 87%. The lambda sign was subsequently identified in none of the 53 pregnancies in which it was absent at 10–14 weeks[12]. Therefore, absence of the lambda sign at 16 or 20 weeks, and presumably thereafter, does not constitute evidence of monochorionicity and consequently does not exclude the possibility of dichorionicity or dizygosity. Conversely, because none of the pregnancies classified as monochorionic at the early scan subsequently developed the lambda sign, the identification of this feature at any stage of pregnancy should be considered as evidence of dichorionicity.

MISCARRIAGE AND PERINATAL MORTALITY

The perinatal mortality rate in twins is around 6 times higher than in singletons[13–17]. This increased mortality, which is mainly due to prematurity-related complications, is higher in monochorionic than dichorionic twin pregnancies. In monochorionic twins, an additional complication to prematurity is twin-to-twin transfusion syndrome. Thus, retrospective studies in which both zygosity and chorionicity were determined after birth reported that the perinatal mortality rate is about 3–4 times higher in monochorionic compared to dichorionic twins, regardless of zygosity[18,19].

A prospective study, in which chorionicity was assessed by ultrasound examination at 10–14 weeks of gestation, compared pregnancy outcome in 102 monochorionic and 365 dichorionic twin pregnancies[20]. There was at least one fetal loss before 24 weeks of gestation in 12.7% of monochorionic and 2.5% of dichorionic pregnancies.

Additionally, there was at least one perinatal loss (at or after 24 weeks) in 4.9% of monochorionic and 2.8% of dichorionic pregnancies[20].

This study confirmed that perinatal mortality in twins, especially those that are monochorionic, is higher than in singleton pregnancies. However, perinatal statistics underestimate the importance of monochorionic placentation to fetal death since the highest rate of mortality is before 24 weeks of gestation (Figure 5)[20]. This hidden mortality confined to monochorionic pregnancies is likely to be the consequence of the underlying chorioangiopagus and severe early-onset twin-to-twin transfusion syndrome. Therefore, reduction of the excess fetal loss in twins, compared to singletons, can only be achieved through early identification of monochorionic pregnancies by ultrasound examination at 11–14 weeks of gestation, and the development of appropriate methods of surveillance and intervention during the second trimester of pregnancy.

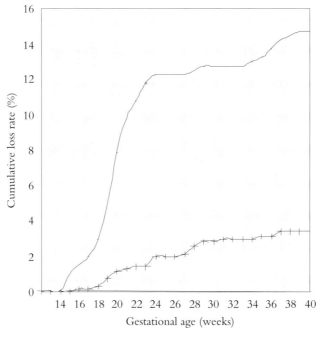

Figure 5   Cumulative fetal loss rates in monochorionic (solid line) and dichorionic (dashed line) twin pregnancies, from 12 weeks of gestation[20]

SEVERE PRETERM DELIVERY

The most important complication of any pregnancy is delivery before term, and especially before 32 weeks. Almost all babies born before 24 weeks die and almost all born after 32 weeks survive. Delivery between 24 and 32 weeks is associated with a high chance of neonatal death and handicap in the survivors. In a singleton pregnancy, the chance of delivery between 24 and 32 weeks is 1–2%. In a study of 467 twin pregnancies in which chorionicity was assessed during the 11–14-week scan, the median gestation at delivery of live births was only marginally earlier in monochorionic (36 weeks), compared to dichorionic (37 weeks) pregnancies[20]. However, the proportion of pregnancies delivering very preterm (before 32 weeks) was nearly twice as high in monochorionic (9.2%) compared to dichorionic (5.5%) twins (Figure 6)[20].

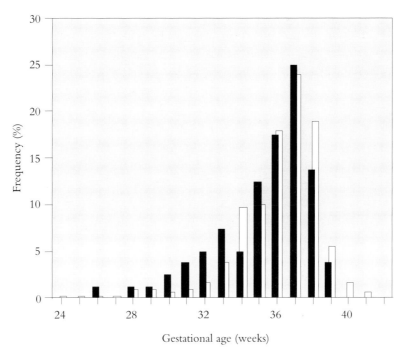

Figure 6 Gestational age distribution at delivery of monochorionic (solid bars) and dichorionic (open bars) twin pregnancies. The proportion of pregnancies delivering very preterm (before 32 weeks) is considerably higher in monochorionic compared to dichorionic twins[20]

The extent to which close monitoring of cervical length and the insertion of cervical sutures in those with a short cervix will reduce the risk of severe preterm delivery remains to be determined.

GROWTH RESTRICTION

In singleton pregnancies, the main factors determining fetal growth are genetic potential and placental function, which is thought to be due mainly to the effectiveness of trophoblastic invasion of the maternal spiral arteries.

In monochorionic twin pregnancies, both the genetic constitution and the factors which govern trophoblastic invasion should be the same for the two fetuses. Consequently, inter-twin disparities in growth are likely to reflect the degree of unequal splitting of the initial single cell mass or the magnitude of imbalance in the bidirectional flow of fetal blood through placental vascular communications between the two circulations. In contrast, since about 90% of dichorionic pregnancies are dizygotic, inter-twin disparities in size would be due to differences in genetic constitution of the fetuses and their placentas.

In twin pregnancies, the risk of delivering growth-restricted babies is about 10 times higher than in singleton pregnancies[21]. In a study of 467 twin pregnancies in which chorionicity was assessed at the 11–14-week scan, the chance of growth restriction (birth weight below the 5th centile for gestation in singletons) of at least one of the fetuses was 34% for monochorionic and 23% for dichorionic twins[20]. Furthermore, the chance of growth restriction of both twins was about four times as high in monochorionic (7.5%) compared to dichorionic (1.7%) pregnancies (Figure 7)[20].

Ultrasonographic studies in the first trimester have examined inter-twin disparities in crown–rump length to determine if this measurement is useful in the prediction of pregnancy outcome. One study examined 180 pregnancies at less than 8 weeks of gestation (median crown–rump length of 8.4 mm) and reported that in those pregnancies resulting in two live births, the median inter-twin disparity in crown–rump length was about 10% (0.9 mm); a difference of more than 3 mm was associated with a 50% chance

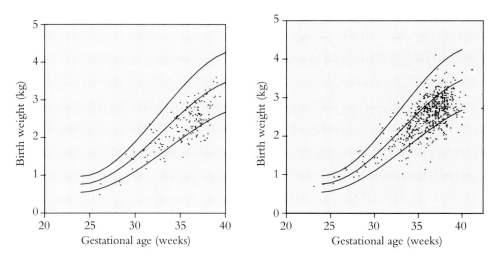

Figure 7 The chance of growth restriction (birth weight below the 5th centile for gestation in singletons) of both twins is about four times as high in monochorionic (left) compared to dichorionic (right) pregnancies[20]

of intrauterine death of the smaller twin[22]. There are also three studies reporting on a total of seven pregnancies discordant for growth restriction or congenital abnormalities that demonstrated large inter-twin disparities in crown–rump length at 6–11 weeks of gestation[23–25].

In a study of 123 monochorionic and 416 dichorionic twin pregnancies, there were no significant differences in inter-twin disparity in crown–rump length at the 11–14-week scan or birth weight between monochorionic and dichorionic twins (Figure 8)[26]. In addition, there was no significant correlation between inter-twin disparities in crown–rump length and inter-twin disparities in birth weight. In dichorionic pregnancies with chromosomally abnormal fetuses, and in those which ended in miscarriage or intrauterine death of one or both fetuses, the inter-twin disparity in crown–rump length was significantly higher than in pregnancies resulting in two live births. However, in the monochorionic twins with adverse pregnancy outcome, there was no significant difference in inter-twin disparity in crown–rump length from pregnancies resulting in two live births[26].

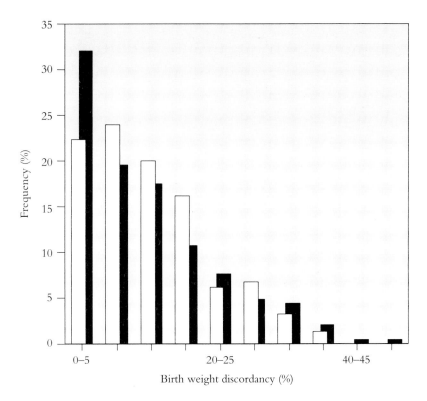

Figure 8   There is no significant inter-twin disparity in birth weight between monochorionic (solid bars) and dichorionic (open bars) twins[26]

In twin pregnancies resulting in live births the median inter-twin disparity in fetal size increases with gestation from about 3% at 12 weeks to 10% at birth[26]. In monochorionic twins, this increasing disparity may be a consequence of the degree of imbalance in fetal nutrition as a result of chronic twin-to-twin transfusion syndrome. Similarly, in dichorionic twins, the increasing disparity in size may also be due to differences in fetal nutrition, but in this case such differences may be a consequence of discordancy in the effectiveness of trophoblastic invasion of the maternal spiral arteries and therefore placental function. The finding, of no significant association between inter-twin disparity in crown–rump length and inter-twin disparity in birth weight[26], suggests that assessment in early pregnancy cannot provide useful prediction of the subsequent development of either mild chronic twin-to-twin transfusion syndrome in monochorionic twins or growth restriction in dichorionic twins.

The findings in dichorionic twins (that adverse pregnancy outcome or chromosomal abnormalities are associated with large inter-twin disparities in crown–rump length)[26], suggest that, in such pregnancies, there is early-onset growth restriction in one of the fetuses, either due to a genetic defect or impaired placentation. In addition, the association between large inter-twin disparities in crown–rump length and miscarriage are compatible with observations that, in multiple pregnancies, spontaneous or iatrogenic death of one of the fetuses can destabilize the whole pregnancy, resulting in miscarriage or severe preterm delivery.

The finding in monochorionic twins, that adverse pregnancy outcome is not associated with large inter-twin disparities in crown–rump length at the 11–14-week scan, suggests that, at this early gestation, fetal growth may not be affected by impaired nutrition through such conditions as chronic fetal hemorrhage. It is possible that at this stage there is programmed fetal growth that may only be affected by serious genetic abnormalities, such as chromosomal defects, or extreme degrees of placental impairment that will subsequently result in fetal death.

TWIN-TO-TWIN TRANSFUSION SYNDROME

In monochorionic twin pregnancies, there are placental vascular anastamoses which allow communication of the two fetoplacental circulations; these anastomoses may be arterio–arterial, veno–venous, or arterio–venous in nature[27]. This phenomenon of a shared circulation between monochorionic twins was first described by Schatz in 1882[28]. Anatomical studies demonstrated that arterio–venous anastomoses are deep in the placenta but almost always proceed through the cotyledonary capillary bed[29]. In about 25% of monochorionic twin pregnancies, imbalance in the net flow of blood across the placental vascular arterio–venous communications from one fetus, the

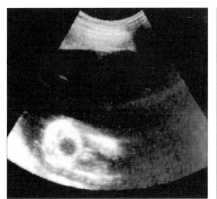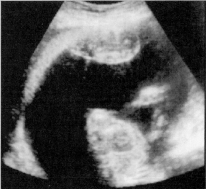

Figure 9 Severe twin-to-twin transfusion syndrome at 20 weeks of gestation. In the polyuric recipient, there is a large bladder and polyhydramnios (left) and the anuric donor is held fixed to the placenta by the collapsed membranes of the anhydramniotic sac (right)

donor, to the other, the recipient, results in twin-to-twin transfusion syndrome; in about half of these cases, there is severe twin-to-twin transfusion syndrome presenting as acute polyhydramnios in the second trimester (Figure 9).

The precise underlying mechanism by which a select population of those mono-chorionic pregnancies with vascular communications go on to develop twin-to-twin transfusion syndrome is not fully understood. However, it has been hypothesized that primary maldevelopment of the placenta of the donor twin may cause increased peripheral resistance in the placental circulation which promotes shunting of blood to the recipient; the donor therefore suffers from both hypovolemia due to blood loss and hypoxia due to placental insufficiency[30,31]. The recipient fetus compensates for its expanded blood volume with polyuria[32], but, since protein and cellular components remain in its circulation, the consequent increase in colloid oncotic pressure draws water from the maternal compartment across the placenta. A vicious cycle of hyper-volemia, polyuria and hyperosmolality is established, leading to high-output heart failure and polyhydramnios.

Traditionally, the diagnosis of twin-to-twin transfusion syndrome was made retrospectively, in the neonatal period, on the basis of an inter-twin difference in birth weight of 20% or more and hemoglobin concentration of 5 g/dl or more[33–35]. These observations were made in live births and therefore the criteria may only apply to relatively mild twin-to-twin transfusion syndrome, since severe cases result in mis-carriage or stillbirth. Additionally, large inter-twin differences in hemoglobin and birth weight are found in some dichorionic twin pregnancies and are not pathognomonic of twin-to-twin transfusion syndrome[36].

Severe disease, with the development of polyhydramnios, becomes apparent at 16–24 weeks of pregnancy. The pathognomonic features of severe twin-to-twin transfusion syndrome by ultrasonographic examination are the presence of a large bladder in the polyuric recipient fetus in the polyhydramniotic sac, and 'absent' bladder in the anuric donor which is found to be 'stuck' and immobile at the edge of the placenta or the uterine wall, where it is held fixed by the collapsed membranes of the anhydramniotic sac (Figure 9). Other sonographic findings that may prove to be of prognostic significance include the presence of a hypertrophic, dilated and dyskinetic heart, with absence or reversal of flow in the ductus venosus during atrial contraction[37]. In the donor, the heart may be dilated, the bowel is hyperechogenic, and there is absent end-diastolic flow in the umbilical artery; these features are commonly seen in hypoxemic fetuses in pregnancies with severe uteroplacental insufficiency. Once the oligohydramnios/polyhydramnios sequence is present, the rate of death of both fetuses is about 90%[31].

Early prediction of twin-to-twin transfusion syndrome

Ultrasonographic features of the underlying hemodynamic changes in severe twin-to-twin transfusion syndrome may be present from as early as 11–14 weeks of gestation and manifest as increased nuchal translucency thickness in one or both of the fetuses. In a study of 132 monochorionic twin pregnancies, including 16 that developed severe twin-to-twin transfusion syndrome at 15–22 weeks of gestation, increased nuchal translucency (above the 95th centile of the normal range) at the 11–14-week scan was associated with a four-fold increase in risk for the subsequent development of severe twin-to-twin transfusion syndrome (Figure 10)[38]. Intertwin discrepancies in crown–rump length were not predictive of subsequent development of twin-to-twin

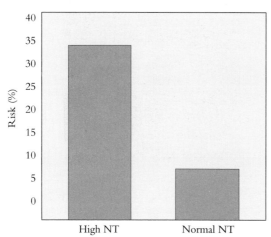

Figure 10 In monochorionic twin pregnancies at the 11–14-week scan, increased nuchal translucency (NT) thickness in one or both fetuses is associated with a four-fold increase in risk for the subsequent development of severe twin-to-twin transfusion syndrome[38]

transfusion syndrome. It is possible that increased nuchal translucency thickness in the recipient fetus may be a manifestation of heart failure due to hypervolemic congestion. With advancing gestation and the development of diuresis that would tend to correct the hypervolemia and reduce heart strain, both the congestive heart failure and nuchal translucency resolve.

In fetuses of monochorionic twin pregnancies, the prevalence of increased nuchal translucency thickness is higher than in dichorionic twins (see section below), presumably because of the circulatory imbalance associated with twin-to-twin transfusion syndrome. Consequently, the presence of increased nuchal translucency thickness in monochorionic twins at 11–14 weeks should stimulate the sonographer to undertake close surveillance for early diagnosis of the clinical features of severe twin-to-twin transfusion syndrome. The extent to which such an earlier diagnosis would lead to therapeutic interventions with a higher survival rate remains to be determined.

An early manifestation of disparity in amniotic fluid volume due to twin-to-twin transfusion syndrome is inter-twin membrane folding, because of the oliguria and collapsed amniotic sac of the donor twin (Figure 11)[39]. In about one-quarter of monochorionic twin pregnancies at 15–17 weeks of gestation, there is membrane folding, and in about half of such cases there is progression to the polyhydramnios/anhydramnios sequence of severe twin-to-twin transfusion syndrome; in the other half, there is moderate twin-to-twin transfusion syndrome with large discrepancies in amniotic fluid volume and fetal size persisting throughout pregnancy. In about 75% of monochorionic twins, there is no membrane fold and these pregnancies are not at increased risk for miscarriage or perinatal death[39].

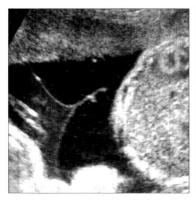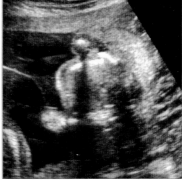

Figure 11   Monochorionic twin pregnancies at 16 weeks of gestation affected by early twin-to-twin transfusion syndrome, showing folding of the inter-twin membrane pointing towards the recipient amniotic sac and the increased echogenicity of the amniotic fluid in the donor sac (left) and folding of the inter-twin membrane around the limb of the donor fetus (right)

In severe twin-to-twin transfusion syndrome presenting with acute polyhydramnios at 16–24 weeks of gestation, survival with expectant management is less than 10%[31]. Improved survival of such pregnancies has been reported after treatment with serial amniocenteses and drainage of large volumes of amniotic fluid; this treatment presumably prevents the polyhydramnios-mediated risk of spontaneous abortion or very premature delivery. In studies published before 1991, amniodrainage was associated with survival in 40–50% of the cases[31]. However, more recent papers have reported survivals of 70–80% of fetuses[40–42].

It is possible that the apparent marked improvement in survival with serial amniodrainage, compared to previous studies that used the same treatment protocols, could, at least in part, be the consequence of the inclusion of pregnancies with moderate twin-to-twin transfusion syndrome. Thus, the widespread use of routine ultrasound examination and the identification of monochorionic pregnancies with large inter-twin disparities in size and amniotic fluid volume could have stimulated obstetricians to undertake amniodrainage in pregnancies with moderate twin-to-twin transfusion syndrome that would have resulted in live births even without such treatment. Since in only about 50% of pregnancies with twin-to-twin transfusion syndrome is the condition severe (where amniodrainage may truly be associated with a survival of about 40–50%), the inclusion of pregnancies with moderate twin-to-twin transfusion syndrome (where survival even with expectant management may be as high as 100%) could account for the apparent recent improvement in survival with amniodrainage from about 40–50% to 70–80%.

MONOAMNIOTIC TWINS

Splitting of the embryonic mass after day 9 of fertilization results in monoamniotic twins. In these cases, there is a single amniotic cavity with a single placenta and the two umbilical cords insert close to each other. Monoamniotic twins are found in about 1% of all twins or about 5% of monochorionic twins. In a series of 1288 twin pregnancies (including 317 monochorionic) examined at the 11–14-week scan at the Harris Birthright Research Centre, King's College Hospital, there were 14 monoamniotic pregnancies (including four with conjoined twins and two with twin reversed arterial perfusion sequence).

In monoamniotic twins, the fetal loss rate is about 50–75%, due to fetal malformations, preterm delivery and complications arising form the close proximity of the two umbilical cords. Cord entanglement is generally thought to be the underlying mechanism for the majority of fetal losses, and attempts have been made to prevent this complication by the administration to the mother of sulindac during the second trimester to stabilize the fetal lie by reducing the amniotic fluid volume[43]. However, cord entaglement is found in most cases of monoamniotic twins and this is usually present from the first trimester of pregnancy[44–46]. Therefore, a more likely cause of fetal death in monoamniotic twins, which occurs suddenly and unpredictably, is acute twin-to-twin transfusion syndrome. The close insertion of the umbilical cords into the placenta is associated with large-caliber anastamoses between the two fetal circulations[46,47]. Consequently, an imbalance in the two circulations could not be sustained for prolonged periods of time (which is necessary for the development of the classic features of twin-to-twin transfusion syndrome), but would rather have major hemodynamic effects, causing sudden fetal death.

On the basis of existing data, the diagnosis of monoamniotic twins at the 11–14-week scan should lead to counselling of the parents as to the high risk of sudden, unexpected and non-preventable fetal death. In our series of eight monoamniotic pregnancies with two separate fetuses diagnosed by the early scan, there were four discordant for major fetal abnormality and these resulted in termination of pregnancy or death of both fetuses. In the four cases where both fetuses were normal, one resulted in survival of both twins, another in survival of one twin and two in intrauterine death of both fetuses (Table 1).

Table 1 Pregnancy outcome and management in eight monoamniotic pregnancies diagnosed at 10–13 weeks of gestation at the Harris Birthright Research Centre

Gestation (weeks)	NT (mm)	Findings	Management	Outcome
13	1.2/1.2	anencephaly/normal	termination	
11	5.5/1.8	body stalk anomaly/normal	termination	
11	4.4/2.0	kyphoscoliosis/normal	termination	
13	6.0/2.0	diaphragmatic hernia/normal	expectant	IUD/IUD at 21 weeks
10	1.7/1.2	normal/normal	expectant	alive/alive at 31 weeks
11	1.1/1.0	normal/normal	expectant	IUD/IUD at 21 weeks
12	2.1/2.1	normal/normal	sulindac	IUD/IUD at 31 weeks
12	1.5/1.5	normal/normal	sulindac	IUD 30 weeks/alive 34 weeks

NT, nuchal translucency thickness; IUD, intrauterine death

Conjoined twins

Splitting of the embryonic mass after day 12 of fertilization results in conjoined twins, which are found in about 1% of monochorionic pregnancies. Conjoined twins are classified, according to the dominant site of interfetal body part connection, into five major types: thoracopagus (thorax, 30–40%), omphalopagus (abdomen, 25–30%), pygopagus (sacrum, 10–20%), ischiopagus (pelvis 6–20%) and craniopagus (head, 2–16%). The prognosis depends on the site and extent of conjoining, but, in general, about 50% are stillborn and one-third of those born alive have severe defects for which surgery is not possible. In the live-born cases in whom planned surgery is carried out, about 60% of infants survive[48,49].

In our four cases of conjoined twins diagnosed at the 11–14-week scan, the nuchal translucency was increased in six of the eight fetuses (0.5 mm and 6.5 mm at 11 weeks, 4.2 mm and 7.5 mm at 11 weeks, 2.4 mm and 3.6 mm at 13 weeks and 3.5 mm and 7.0 mm at 13 weeks, respectively). However, the extent to which nuchal translucency provides useful prediction as to the outcome of such pregnancies is uncertain. In cases diagnosed in the first trimester, the patients usually elect termination of pregnancy. There are no series reporting on the natural history of the condition.

Twin reversed arterial perfusion sequence

The most extreme manifestation of twin-to-twin transfusion syndrome, found in approximately 1% of monochorionic twin pregnancies, is acardiac twinning (acardius chorioangiopagus parasiticus). This twin disorder has been named 'twin reversed arterial perfusion' (TRAP) sequence because the underlying mechanism is thought to be disruption of normal vascular perfusion and development of one twin (the recipient) due to an umbilical arterio–arterio anastomosis with the other (donor or pump) twin[50]. At least 50% of donor twins die due to congestive heart failure or severe preterm delivery, the consequence of polyhydramnios[50,51]. All perfused twins die due to the associated multiple malformations.

Prenatal treatment is by occlusion of the blood flow to the acardiac twin by endoscopic ligation or laser coagulation of the umbilical cord[52,53]. A less invasive technique is ultrasound-guided laser coagulation of the umbilical cord vessels within the abdomen of the acardiac twin, which is carried out at about 16 weeks of gestation.

DEATH OF ONE FETUS IN TWIN PREGNANCY

Intrauterine death of a fetus in a twin pregnancy may be associated with adverse outcome for the co-twin, but the type and degree of risk are dependent on the chorionicity of the pregnancy.

Missed abortions in twin pregnancies in the first trimester

In singleton pregnancies at the 11–14-week scan, the prevalence of missed abortion is about 2%[54]. In a study of 492 twin pregnancies, the prevalence of death of one or both of the fetuses at the early scan was 5%; additionally, in 24% of pregnancies with one fetal death, there was a subsequent death of the co-twin or miscarriage[55]. In twin pregnancies with two live fetuses at 10–14 weeks, the overall risk of subsequent miscarriage is about 5% (2% for dichorionic and 12% for monochorionic pregnancies). Therefore, the prevalence of missed abortion at the 11–14-week scan in twin pregnancies is about twice as high as in singletons and the risk of subsequent miscarriage in twins with one missed abortion is about five times as high as in normal twins.

Intrauterine death of one fetus in the second or third trimester

Death of one fetus in dichorionic pregnancies carries a risk to the remaining fetus, mainly due to preterm delivery, which may be the consequence of release of cytokines and prostaglandins by the resorbing dead placenta. In dichorionic twins, the risk of death or handicap of the co-twin in such cases is about 5–10%, whereas, in monochorionic twins, there is at least a 25% risk of death or neurological handicap due to hypotensive episodes in addition to the risk of preterm delivery[56]. The acute hypotensive episode is the result of hemorrhage from the live fetus into the dead fetoplacental unit[57,58]. In singleton pregnancies, death and retention of the fetus may be associated with maternal disseminated intravascular coagulation; however, in twin pregnancies with one dead fetus, this complication has only rarely been reported.

STRUCTURAL DEFECTS IN MULTIPLE PREGNANCY

Fetal structural defects in twin pregnancies can be grouped into those which also occur in singletons and those specific to the twinning process, the latter being unique to monozygotic twins. For any given defect, the pregnancy may be concordant or discordant in terms of both the presence or type of abnormality and its severity. There is no increased risk of congenital abnormalities in pregnancies from assisted reproduction compared to those achieved spontaneously[59].

Discordancies in dizygotic twins are usually due to differences in genetic predisposition. In monozygotic pregnancies discordancies may be:

(1) The consequence of variation in gene expression (secondary to postzygotic mutation, parenteral imprinting effects or asymmetric X-inactivation);

(2) Asymmetric splitting of the cell mass, in either volume or cytoplasmic content, resulting in unequal potential for development (the 'Christmas cracker' hypothesis);

(3) Splitting after laterality gradients are determined, resulting in malformations of laterality, such as cardiac and mid-line defects; or

(4) Hemodynamic factors in monochorionic pregnancies resulting in abnormal flow patterns, and thence in cardiac defects or the twin reversed arterial perfusion sequence.

The prevalence of structural defects per fetus in dizygotic twins is the same as in singletons, whereas the rate in monozygotic twins is 2–3 times higher[60,61]. Concordance of defects (both fetuses being affected) is uncommon, being found in about 10% of dichorionic and 20% of monochorionic pregnancies.

Management of pregnancies discordant for structural defects

Multiple pregnancies discordant for a fetal abnormality can essentially be managed expectantly or by selective fetocide of the abnormal twin. In cases where the abnormality is non-lethal but may well result in serious handicap, the parents need to decide whether the potential burden of a handicapped child is enough to risk loss of the normal twin from fetocide-related complications. In cases where the abnormality is lethal, it may be best to avoid such risk to the normal fetus, unless the condition itself threatens the survival of the normal twin.

This management dilemma is exemplified by pregnancies discordant for anencephaly, which is always lethal but may be associated with the development of polyhydramnios, which places the normal co-twin at risk of neonatal death from severe preterm delivery.

A study of 24 twin pregnancies discordant for anencephaly reported that 13 were dichorionic and 11 monochorionic[62]. In the dichorionic group, five pregnancies had selective fetocide at 17–21 weeks; one pregnancy resulted in spontaneous abortion but, in the others, a healthy baby was delivered at a median gestation of 37 weeks. The other eight dichorionic pregnancies were managed expectantly but three developed polyhydramnios at 26–30 weeks; in one case amniodrainage and in another selective fetocide were carried out. In this group, the median gestation at delivery was 35 weeks. The 11 monochorionic pregnancies were managed expectantly and, in three, there was intrauterine death of both fetuses. In the other eight cases, the normal twin was liveborn at a median gestation of 34 weeks; in four of the pregnancies, polyhydramnios developed and two of these were managed by amniodrainage.

The main issues in the management of pregnancies discordant for anencephaly are:

(1) The prevalences of monochorionicity and dichorionicity in twin pregnancies discordant for anencephaly are similar, and, by implication, the prevalence of anencephaly is much higher in monochorionic than dichorionic pregnancies. In a study of 2874 twin and 334 912 singleton pregnancies from the same population over the same period, the prevalence of anencephaly was 10.4/10 000 in twins compared to 2.8/10 000 in singletons[63]. This increase was mainly found in like-sex compared to unlike-sex pairs and, by implication, in monozygotic compared to dizygotic pregnancies. Furthermore, the prevalence of concordancy for anencephaly in monozygotic twins is twice as high as in dizygotic pregnancies[64], and, consequently, there may be a genetic contribution to the pathogenesis of neural tube defects; however, concordancy for anencephaly is found in less than 10% of affected pregnancies and, therefore, the contribution of environmental factors may be of greater importance than that of genetic factors.

(2) Anencephaly is associated with a high risk of preterm delivery before 32 weeks, which is usually due to the development of polyhydramnios secondary to reduced fetal swallowing. In a study of 60 singleton pregnancies with anencephaly, before the advent of prenatal diagnosis, the prevalence of clinical polyhydramnios was 49%[65].

(3) In dichorionic twins discordant for anencephaly, the two management options are selective fetocide or serial ultrasound examinations for early diagnosis of polyhydramnios, which can then be treated either by amniodrainage or selective fetocide. Selective fetocide is associated with mortality of the normal twin through procedure-related miscarriage. The risk of miscarriage after selective fetocide is about 5% or 15% depending on whether the procedure is carried out before or after 16 weeks of gestation, respectively[66]. Since first-trimester ultrasound examination is increasingly being introduced as part of routine antenatal care and anencephaly can be reliably diagnosed at 11–14 weeks of gestation[67], it is possible that the majority of twin pregnancies discordant for anencephaly will now be diagnosed sufficiently early for safer selective fetocide. An additional advantage of earlier selective fetocide is that the risk of severe preterm delivery is reduced and, on average, the gestation at delivery of the normal twin is later than with fetocide after 16 weeks[66].

(4) In monochorionic twin pregnancies, selective fetocide is not possible because death of the anencephalic fetus would be followed by death of the normal co-twin; this may be due to transplacental passage of the injected potassium chloride or acute exsanguination through the vascular anastomoses into the placenta of the dead anencephalic fetus. However, since expectant management is associated with spontaneous intrauterine death of the anencephalic fetus in about 25% of cases, this option can also result in the death of the normal twin through similar mechanisms. Future research may demonstrate that the optimal management of monochorionic twin pregnancies discordant for anencephaly is selective fetocide by occlusion of the umbilical cord vessels of the abnormal fetus.

In twin pregnancies discordant for lethal abnormalities, the aims are to maximize the chances of survival of the normal twin and prevent severe preterm delivery. Early diagnosis through routine ultrasound examination at 11–14 weeks will inevitably stimulate further research in this area. The questions to be resolved by multicenter randomized studies are whether the risk of death and severe preterm delivery are less with expectant management or selective fetocide in the first trimester. In the case of dichorionic pregnancies, fetocide can be carried out by the traditional method of intracardiac injection of potassium chloride, whereas, in monochorionic pregnancies, fetocide would necessitate occlusion of the umbilical cord vessels.

CHROMOSOMAL DEFECTS IN MULTIPLE PREGNANCY

In multiple pregnancies compared to singletons, prenatal diagnosis of chromosomal abnormalities is complicated because, first, effective methods of screening, such as maternal serum biochemistry, are not applicable; second, the techniques of invasive testing may provide uncertain results or may be associated with higher risks of miscarriage; and, third, the fetuses may be discordant for an abnormality, in which case one of the options for the subsequent management of the pregnancy is selective fetocide.

Screening for chromosomal defects

In dizygotic pregnancies, the maternal age-related risk for chromosomal abnormalities for each twin may be the same as in singleton pregnancies and, therefore, the chance that at least one fetus is affected by a chromosomal defect is twice as high as in singleton pregnancies. Furthermore, since the rate of dizygotic twinning increases with maternal age, the proportion of twin pregnancies with chromosomal defects is higher than in singleton pregnancies.

In monozygotic twins, the risk for chromosomal abnormalities is the same as in singleton pregnancies and, in the vast majority of cases, both fetuses are affected. There are, however, occasional case reports of monozygotic twins discordant for abnormalities of autosomes or sex chromosomes, most commonly with one fetus having Turner syndrome and the other either a normal male or female phenotype, but usually with a mosaic karyotype[68–71].

The relative proportion of spontaneous dizygotic to monozygotic twins in the United Kingdom is about 2:1 and, therefore, the prevalence of chromosomal abnormalities affecting at least one fetus in twin pregnancies would be expected to be about 1.6 times that in singletons.

Since it is now possible to determine chorionicity antenatally by ultrasonography, in counselling parents, it is possible to give more specific estimates of one and/or both fetuses being affected, depending on chorionicity. Thus, in monochorionic twins, the parents can be counselled that both fetuses would be affected and this risk is similar to that in singleton pregnancies. If the pregnancy is dichorionic, then the parents can be counselled that the risk of discordancy for a chromosomal abnormality is about twice that in singleton pregnancies, whereas the risk that both fetuses would be affected can be derived by squaring the singleton risk ratio. For example, in a 40-year-old woman with a risk for trisomy 21 of about 1 in 100 based on maternal age, in a dizygotic twin pregnancy the risk that one fetus would be affected would be 1 in 50 (1 in 100 plus 1 in 100), whereas the risk that both fetuses would be affected is 1 in 10,000 (1 in 100 × 1 in 100). This is, in reality, an oversimplification, since, unlike monochorionic pregnancies that are always monozygotic, only about 90% of dichorionic pregnancies are dizygotic.

Screening by second-trimester biochemistry

In singleton pregnancies, screening for trisomy 21 by a combination of maternal age and second-trimester maternal serum biochemistry can detect about 60% of trisomy 21 cases for a 5% false-positive rate.

In twin pregnancies, the median values for maternal serum markers, such as α-fetoprotein, hCG, free β-hCG and inhibin-A, are about twice those for singleton pregnancies[72]. When this is taken into account in the mathematical modelling for calculation of risks, it is estimated that serum screening in twins may identify about 45% of affected fetuses for a 5% false-positive rate[72].

Even if prospective studies demonstrate that serum testing in twins is effective, the following problems would still need to be addressed:

(1) The detection rate for an acceptable low false-positive rate, especially since invasive testing in multiple pregnancies is technically more demanding;

(2) In the presence of a 'screen-positive' result, there is no feature to suggest which fetus may be affected; and

(3) If the pregnancy is discordant for a chromosomal defect, further management by way of selective termination carries increased risk in the second compared to the first trimester.

Screening by first-trimester biochemistry

In a prospective screening study by measurement of fetal nuchal translucency thickness, maternal serum free β-hCG was measured in 4181 singleton and 148 twin pregnancies; in the latter group, there were 12 pregnancies with trisomy 21 in either one ($n = 10$) or both ($n = 2$) fetuses[73]. In the normal twin pregnancies, compared to singletons, the median maternal serum free β-hCG adjusted for maternal weight was 1.94 MoM. In the 12 trisomy 21 twin pregnancies, the median level of free β-hCG was significantly higher than in normal twins but the level was above the 95th centile in only one case. These results suggest that measurement of maternal serum free β-hCG is unlikely to be useful in the prediction of fetal trisomy 21 at 11–14 weeks.

Screening by fetal nuchal translucency thickness

In a screening study for trisomy 21 involving 448 twin pregnancies, nuchal translucency thickness was measured in each fetus and the risk was estimated by combining with maternal age. The nuchal translucency was above the 95th centile of the normal range (for crown–rump length in singletons) in 7.3% fetuses, including 88% of those with trisomy 21 (Table 2)[74]. Increased translucency was also present in four fetuses with other chromosomal abnormalities. In the chromosomally normal twin pregnancies, the prevalence of increased nuchal translucency was higher in fetuses of monochorionic than dichorionic pregnancies. The minimum estimated risk for trisomy 21, based on maternal age and fetal nuchal translucency thickness, was 1 in 300 in 19.5% of the twins, including all eight of those with trisomy 21[74].

These findings suggest that, in dichorionic twin pregnancies, the sensitivity and false- positive rate of fetal nuchal translucency thickness in screening for trisomy 21 are similar to those in singleton pregnancies. Therefore, effective screening and diagnosis of major chromosomal abnormalities can be achieved in the first trimester, allowing the

Table 2 Prevalence of fetal nuchal translucency thickness (NT) above the 95th centile (for crown–rump length in singletons), in singleton, monochorionic twin pregnancies and dichorionic twin pregnancies[74]

	Fetuses with increased NT	Pregnancies with increased NT in at least one of the fetuses	Pregnancies with increased NT in both fetuses
Singleton	1122 (5.2%)	—	—
Twin (n = 448)	65 (7.3%)	52 (11.6%)	13 (2.9%)
Monochorionic (n = 95)	16 (8.4%)	13 (13.7%)	3 (3.2%)
Dichorionic (n = 353)	49 (6.9%)	39 (11.1%)	10 (2.8%)

possibility of earlier and therefore safer selective fetocide for those parents that choose this option.

In monochorionic pregnancies (unlike dichorionic twins), the false-positive rate of nuchal translucency screening is higher than in singletons. In monochorionic pregnancies, increased nuchal translucency in one of the fetuses should not lead to the erroneous conclusion of discordant risk for a chromosomal abnormality, but rather should stimulate the search for alternative causes, such as twin-to-twin transfusion syndrome.

In an extended series of 303 monochorionic pregnancies examined at the Harris Birthright Research Centre at King's College Hospital, the nuchal translucency was above the 95th centile in 52 (8.6%) of the 606 fetuses, and in at least one fetus in 41 (13.5%) of the 303 pregnancies. There were two cases of both fetuses being affected by trisomy 21; in one case, the nuchal translucency was increased in both fetuses (3.1 mm and 2.4 mm at 11 weeks), but in the second case the translucency was increased only in one of the fetuses (8.2 mm and 1.8 mm at 13 weeks). The number of cases examined is still too small to draw definite conclusions as to whether, in the calculation of risk of trisomy 21 in monochorionic pregnancies, the nuchal translucency of the fetus with the largest or the smallest measurement (or the average of the two) should be considered.

Fetal karyotyping in twins

Fetal karyotyping requires invasive testing by amniocentesis or chorionic villus sampling. In singleton pregnancies, both techniques are highly successful in providing samples for cytogenetic analysis and the risk of fetal loss from the two procedures is similar (about 1% above the background risk). Therefore, in singleton pregnancies, the method of choice for fetal karyotyping may be chorionic villus sampling because of the advantages of early diagnosis, namely earlier reassurance for the majority of parents that

171

the fetal karyotype is normal and the option of earlier termination for the few with an affected pregnancy.

In twin pregnancies, selection of the appropriate invasive technique depends on the:

(1) Accuracy of obtaining a result from both fetuses;

(2) Procedure-related risk of fetal loss; and

(3) The risks of selective fetocide should the pregnancy be found to be discordant for an abnormality and the parents choose this option.

Amniocentesis in twins can be carried out through a single uterine entry (Figure 12). It is effective in providing a reliable karyotype for both fetuses and the procedure may be as safe as in singleton pregnancies[75]. However, cytogenetic results are not available until around 18 weeks and the risk of miscarriage after selective fetocide at this gestation is three times higher than with fetocide before 16 weeks[66].

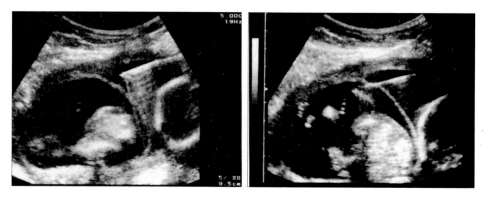

Figure 12 Amniocentesis in twins using the single-needle technique. A 20-gauge needle with a stylet is guided into one amniotic sac (left). After aspiration of 10 ml of amniotic fluid, the syringe is removed, the stylet is replaced, and the needle is advanced through the inter-twin membrane under continuous ultrasound guidance into the second sac (right). The stylet is then removed and amniotic fluid aspirated; the first 1 ml is discarded to avoid possible contamination with fluid from the first sac

Chorionic villus sampling can be carried out in multiple pregnancies but, in about 5% of cases, there is uncertainty if both placentas have been sampled, especially in cases where the placentas are on the same side of the uterus[76–79]. To ensure that both fetuses are karyotyped, the extreme ends of the placentas should be reached through a single uterine entry of one needle, or two separate needle insertions are necessary; therefore the procedure-related risk of miscarriage may be higher than with amniocentesis. The advantage of chorionic villus sampling is that it provides results sufficiently early to allow for safer selective fetocide.

The choice of invasive technique in twins should therefore be based on the use of individual risk calculated by maternal age and fetal nuchal translucency thickness[80]. When the risk for chromosomal defect in at least one of the fetuses is high (more than 1 in 50), it may be preferable to perform chorionic villus sampling. For pregnancies with a lower risk, amniocentesis at 16 weeks would be the favorite option.

There is an additional advantage of screening by measurement of nuchal translucency thickness in this context; when there is discordancy for a chromosomal abnormality, the presence of a sonographically detectable marker (increased nuchal translucency) helps to ensure the correct identification of the abnormal twin should the parents choose selective termination.

Management of twin pregnancies discordant for chromosomal abnormalities

In a study of 27 twin pregnancies affected by fetal trisomies, there were seven cases where both fetuses were trisomic and in these the parents opted for termination of pregnancy; termination was also performed in another pregnancy where one fetus had trisomy 18 and the chromosomally normal co-twin had a major facial cleft[81]. In 19 cases, one fetus had either trisomy 21 ($n = 14$) or trisomy 18 ($n = 5$) and the other was normal. Selective fetocide was carried out in 13 of the 14 pregnancies discordant for trisomy 21 and in one of the five with trisomy 18. In the four cases discordant for trisomy 18 that were managed expectantly, the trisomic baby died *in utero* or in the neonatal period, whereas the normal co-twin was liveborn at 33–40 (median 37) weeks. In the 14 cases of selective fetocide, the chromosomally normal co-twin was live born at 24–41 (median 38) weeks of gestation and there was an inverse relationship between the gestation at fetocide and gestation at delivery [81].

The main issues in the management of twin pregnancies with fetal trisomies are:

(1) When both fetuses are chromosomally abnormal, the parents usually choose termination of pregnancy.

(2) In pregnancies discordant for chromosomal abnormalities, the main options are either selective fetocide or expectant management. In such cases, the decision is essentially based on the relative risk of selective fetocide causing miscarriage and hence death of the normal baby, compared to the potential burden of caring for a handicapped child.

(3) Selective fetocide can result in spontaneous abortion or severe preterm delivery, which may occur several months after the procedure. The risk for these complications is related to the gestation at fetocide; selective fetocide after 16 weeks of gestation is associated with a three-fold increase in risk compared to reduction before 16 weeks, and there is an inverse correlation between the gestation at fetocide with the gestation at delivery[66]. In embryo reduction of multifetal pregnancies, there is an increase in maternal serum α-fetoprotein which is proportional to the number of dead fetuses and this increase persists for 8–12 weeks, when there is complete resorption of the dead fetoplacental tissue[82]. It is possible that the resorbing dead fetoplacental tissue triggers an intrauterine inflammatory process, which is proportional to the amount of dead tissue and therefore the gestation at fetocide. Such an inflammatory process could result in the release of cytokines and prostaglandins which would, in turn, induce uterine activity with consequent miscarriage/ preterm labor.

(4) In pregnancies discordant for trisomy 21, the usual choice is selective fetocide, because with expectant management the majority of affected babies would survive. In the case of trisomy 18, about 85% of affected fetuses die *in utero* and those that are liveborn usually die within the first year of life. In this respect, expectant management may be the preferred option; this would certainly avoid the procedure-related complications from selective fetocide. The alternative view is that the amount of dead fetoplacental tissue (and therefore the risk for consequent miscarriage or preterm labor) would be less after fetocide at 12 weeks rather than after spontaneous death of the trisomy 18 fetus at a later stage of pregnancy.

PRENATAL DETERMINATION OF CHORIONICITY

In twin pregnancies, prenatal diagnosis of chorionicity is important because:

(1) Chorionicity, rather than zygosity, is the main factor determining pregnancy outcome. In monochorionic twins, the rates of miscarriage and perinatal death are much higher than in dichorionic twins. This increase in risk has been attributed to complications arising from the shared placental circulation, which is confined to monochorionic twins.

(2) Death of a monochorionic fetus is associated with a high chance of sudden death or severe neurological impairment in the co-twin, which is important both for parental counselling should this occur spontaneously and for the management of discordant fetal abnormality.

(3) Diagnostic testing of patients at high risk for genetic disorders and chromosomal abnormalities is dependent on chorionicity. In monochorionic twin pregnancies, when undertaking invasive diagnostic tests such as amniocentesis or chorionic villus sampling, it may be unnecessary to sample both fetuses since they are monozygotic and, therefore, have identical genetic compositions.

(4) In the management of a twin pregnancy discordant for a major fetal defect, one of the options is selective fetocide, but in monochorionic twins this procedure should be avoided, otherwise both fetuses could die or the survivor could suffer severe neurological impairment.

(5) In patients who did not have accurate determination of chorionicity in the first trimester but are subsequently found to have the 'lambda' sign present, the pregnancy can be considered to be in a lower-risk category for subsequent miscarriage or perinatal death. Furthermore, if the parents request invasive prenatal diagnosis of genetic syndromes and chromosomal defects, both twins should be sampled because such pregnancies are usually dizygotic. Since these pregnancies are dichorionic, one of the options to be considered in cases with discordant fetal malformations can be selective fetocide. In contrast, absence of the 'lambda' sign at 16–20 weeks does not exclude dizygosity. Therefore, invasive prenatal diagnosis should still involve sampling of both fetuses. However, in terms of management for discordant fetal malformation, these pregnancies must be considered monochorionic, and hence selective fetocide is precluded because, due to the shared placental circulation if the pregnancy is truly monochorionic, fetocide may result in death or neurological impairment of the healthy twin. In the absence of the lambda sign, selective fetocide can only be considered as an option if the placentas are separate or the twins are proven to be dizygotic, by the sonographic demonstration of discordant fetal sexes or by the presence of different genetic markers through examination of amniotic fluid or fetal blood.

MULTIFETAL PREGNANCY AND EMBRYO REDUCTION

An adverse consequence of the widespread introduction of assisted reproductive techniques has been an exponential increase in the prevalence of multifetal pregnancies[13]. Such pregnancies are associated with increased risk of miscarriage and perinatal death[83]. In addition, there is increased risk of handicap. A study of births in Western Australia from 1980 to 1989 reported that the prevalence of cerebral palsy (per 1000 survivors up to 1 year of age) was 1.6 for singletons, 7.3 for twins and 28 for triplets[84]. Similarly, a study of 705 twin pairs (1410 twins), 96 sets of triplets (287 triplets excluding one infant death) and seven sets of quadruplets (27 quadruplets excluding one infant death) reported that the prevalence of cerebral palsy (per 1000 survivors) was 9 in twins, 31 in triplets and 111 in quadruplets[85]. The risk of cerebral palsy was mainly related to preterm delivery and therefore the chance for the parents that their pregnancy would result in at least one child with cerebral palsy was 1.5%, 8.0% and 42.9% in twin, triplet, and quadruplet pregnancies, respectively.

One of the options in the management of multifetal pregnancies is embryo reduction to twins, which is associated with a reduction in the background risk of adverse pregnancy outcome.

Technique and timing of embryo reduction

Iatrogenic fetal death is achieved by the ultrasound-guided injection of potassium chloride in the fetal heart or thorax. During the 3–4 months following reduction, there is gradual resorption of the dead fetuses and their placentas. It is technically feasible to perform reduction from as early as 7 weeks and the earlier the gestation the smaller the dead fetoplacental tissue mass, with the theoretical advantage of a lower rate of miscarriage. However, it is preferable that the procedure is delayed until 11–13 weeks to allow for spontaneous reduction. Furthermore, at this gestation, it is possible to diagnose major fetal abnormalities and also, through measurement of nuchal translucency thickness, to screen for chromosomal defects. If all fetuses appear to be normal, the ones chosen for reduction are those furthest away from the cervix to avoid the potential risk of amniorrhexis and ascending infection from the lower genital track. Ultrasound examination is also essential for the determination of chorionicity. In dichorionic triplets, selective fetocide of one of the monochorionic pair may lead to death or neurological sequelae in the co-twin, whereas iatrogenic death of the fetus with a separate placenta will result in a monochorionic twin pregnancy that is associated with a much higher risk of miscarriage or severe preterm delivery than dichorionic twins. Consequently, the parents may choose to convert the pregnancy into a singleton one by fetocide of both monochorionic twins.

Results of multifetal pregnancy reduction

The largest series combining data from nine centers throughout the world includes 1789 pregnancies undergoing fetal reduction from a mean starting number of four (two to more than six fetuses) to a finishing number of two (range 1–3) fetuses[86]. In 11.7% of cases, there was miscarriage before 24 weeks, in 13.3% severe preterm delivery at 24–32 weeks, and in 75.0% delivery was beyond 32 weeks. The miscarriage rate and severe preterm delivery rate were related to both the starting and finishing number of fetuses.

Gestation at delivery, birth weight and pregnancy outcome of surviving fetuses from 127 multifetal pregnancies (3–8, median 4 fetuses) undergoing embryo reduction to twins were compared to 354 chromosomally normal non-reduced dichorionic twin pregnancies[87]. In multifetal pregnancies reduced to twins, compared to the non-reduced twins, there was a five-fold increase in risk of miscarriage before 24 weeks (12.6% compared to 2.5%), a doubling of risk of severe preterm delivery before 33 weeks (17.1% compared to 7.6%) and a small reduction in birth weight for gestation (deficit of 0.94 SDs compared to 0.65 SDs). Furthermore, the interval between embryo reduction and miscarriage or delivery was associated with the gestation at reduction, which presumably reflects the amount of dead fetoplacental tissue.

Miscarriage within 2 weeks of embryo reduction is about 2%, which is similar to that of early amniocentesis in singleton pregnancies[87,88]. Therefore, most miscarriages associated with multifetal pregnancy reduction are not due to the needling involved in reduction.

The most likely cause of pregnancy loss and severe preterm delivery in multifetal pregnancies following reduction is the development of an inflammatory response to the resorbing dead fetoplacental tissue, with subsequent release of cytokines and stimulation of prostaglandins. High levels of α-fetoprotein are found in the amniotic fluid of twin pregnancies after the spontaneous death of one of the fetuses and in multifetal pregnancies after reduction[89–91]. Similarly, both spontaneous fetal death and disruption in the fetoplacental barrier are associated with high maternal serum α-fetoprotein levels[92,93]. It has been previously reported that, in multifetal pregnancies, following the iatrogenic death of fetuses there is an increase in maternal serum α-fetoprotein concentration that is proportional to the amount of dead fetoplacental tissue and this increase persists for several months following the procedure[82].

The main difference between the reduced and non-reduced pregnancies was miscarriage or severe preterm delivery up to 33 weeks. This finding is compatible with the hypothesis of a trigger of labor arising from the resorption of necrotic tissue, since the risk of early delivery was related to the gestation at reduction, and therefore the size of the dead fetoplacental units. An alternative mechanism of preterm delivery is the decline of hormonal support to the pregnancy following pregnancy reduction. Multifetal pregnancy reduction to twins is associated with a relative decrease in maternal serum concentrations of placental hormones, such as human chorionic gonadotropin, progesterone and estriol, which occurs within 2 weeks of the reduction and persists for at least 3 months[94].

Another possible explanation for fetal loss after reduction, as well as the finding that in multifetal pregnancies reduced to twins the birth weight for gestation is smaller than in non-reduced twins, is that, in the human, the maximum capacity of the endometrium/decidua to maintain a pregnancy is achieved with twins. In multifetal pregnancies, there is crowding and each fetal–placental–endometrial unit has less potential for growth and development than in twin pregnancies. After embryo reduction, the surviving twins have smaller placental units and therefore remain at a disadvantage compared to natural twins and this is manifested as spontaneous abortion, severe preterm delivery or growth restriction. Supportive evidence for this hypothesis is provided by changes in the maternal blood levels of placental protein 14 (PP14) and insulin-like growth factor binding protein-1 (IGFBP-1), which are the major protein products of the decidua of early pregnancy. Maternal plasma IGFBP-1 and PP14 concentrations in twin pregnancies are higher than those in singletons but the levels are not further increased with larger numbers of fetuses. In multifetal pregnancies reduced to twins, maternal serum concentrations of IGFBP-1 and PP14 decrease to levels characteristic of singleton rather than non-reduced twin pregnancies[95].

Reduction from trichorionic triplets to twins

In higher-order multifetal pregnancies, there is evidence that embryo reduction to twins is associated with a decrease in the background risk of perinatal death and handicap. However, in the case of triplet pregnancies reduced to twins, compared to those managed expectantly, the chance of survival is not improved but the risk of handicap may be lower.

Data from studies reporting on gestation at recruitment, and rates of miscarriage and severe preterm delivery in reduced and non-reduced triplet pregnancies (Table 3)[96–113] suggest that fetal reduction to twins is associated with a significantly higher rate of miscarriage (8.3% versus 3.5%), but a 3-fold reduction in severe preterm delivery rate (20.5% versus 6.9%).

On the basis of these results and also the gestational age distribution of reduced and non-reduced triplet pregnancies delivering at 24–31 weeks[102,105,113], and the survival and handicap rates of singleton pregnancies of the same gestational age[114], it was estimated that:

(1) In trichorionic triplets managed expectantly, the survival probability is 92.4% with a 95.8% chance that at least one baby will be born alive and a 2.1% chance that at least one will be handicapped[105].

Table 3 Studies reporting on outcome of triplet pregnancies managed with and without embryo reduction to twins. The studies included are those which provide data on gestation at recruitment and allow calculation of the rates of miscarriage and severe preterm delivery

Author	n	Gestation at recruitment/ reduction (weeks)	Miscarriage at < 24 weeks	Delivery at < 32 weeks
Without embryo reduction				
Lipitz et al. 1989[96]	78	20*	—	20/78
Kingsland et al. 1990[97]	43	16*	—	5/43
Seoud et al. 1991[98]	26	6–8†	2/26	—
Melgar et al. 1991[99]	20	9–14†	0/20	—
Porreco et al. 1991[100]	11	10–11	0/11	1/11
Bollen et al. 1993[101]	39	7	2/39	9/37
Macones et al. 1993[102]	14	16	0/14	6/14
Check et al. 1993[103]	23	9–13	0/23	2/23
Boulot et al. 1993[104]	48	8–13	3/48	7/45
Sebire et al. 1997[105]	47	8–13	1/47	11/46
Total		10 (6–14)	8/228 (3.5%)	61/297 (20.5%)
With embryo reduction				
Porreco et al. 1991[100]	13	10–11	1/13	1/12
Melgar et al. 1991[99]	5	9–14†	0/5	—
Vauthier-Brouzes et al. 1992[106]	14	10–12	0/14	2/14
Boulot et al. 1993[104]	32	8–13	4/32	2/28
Check et al. 1993[103]	6	9–13	0/6	0/6
Macones et al. 1993[102]	47	9–12	4/47	3/43
Bollen et al. 1993[101]	33	7	3/33	1/30
Timor-Tritsch et al. 1993[107]	43	9–10†	6/43	—
Lynch et al. 1990[108] Berkowitz et al. 1993[109]	88	10–13	7/88	4/81
Tabsh 1990, 1993[110,111]	66	11–13†	4/66	—
Shalev et al. 1989[112] Lipitz et al. 1994[113]	34	10–13	3/34	3/31
Sebire et al. 1997[105]	66	7–13	5/66	5/61
Total		10 (7–14)	37/447 (8.3%)	21/306 (6.9%)

*Data from these studies were used only for the calculation of gestation at delivery not miscarriage rates; †data from these studies were used only for the calculation of miscarriage rates not gestation at delivery

(2) In triplets reduced to twins, the survival probability is 89.7% with a 91.4% chance that at least one baby will be born alive and a 0.5% chance that at least one will be handicapped[105].

On the basis of currently available data, parents can be counselled that, in trichorionic triplet pregnancies, with all three fetuses being alive at 12 weeks of gestation, the rates of miscarriage and delivery before 32 weeks are about 4% and 20%, respectively. Furthermore, in triplets reduced to twins, there is an increase in miscarriage rate to about 8% but a decrease in the rate of severe preterm delivery to 10%[105]. Irrespective of the chosen management, there is a more than 90% chance of live births and the potential risk of severe handicap in the survivors is about 1–3%.

REFERENCES

1. Edwards RG, Mettler L, Walters DE. Identical twins and in vitro fertilization. *J In Vitro Fertil Embryo Transf* 1986;3:114–17

2. Alikani M, Noyes N, Cohen J, Rosenwaks Z. Monozygotic twinning in the human is associated with the zona pellucida architecture. *Hum Reprod* 1994;9:1318–21

3. Derom C, Vlietinck R, Derom R, Van Den Berghe H, Thiery M. Increased monozygotic twinning rate after ovulation induction. *Lancet* 1987;1:1236–8

4. Winn HN, Gabrielli S, Reece EA, Roberts JA, Salafia C, Hobbins JC. Ultrasonographic criteria for the prenatal diagnosis of placental chorionicity in twin gestations. *Am J Obstet Gynecol* 1989;161;1540–2

5. Stagiannis KD, Sepulveda W, Southwell D, Price DA, Fisk NM. Ultrasonographic measurement of the dividing membrane in twin pregnancy during the second and third trimesters: a reproducibility study. *Am J Obstet Gynecol* 1995;173:1546–50

6. Kurtz AB, Wapner RJ, Mata J, Johnson A, Morgan P. Twin pregnancies: accuracy of first-trimester abdominal US in predicting chorionicity and amnionicity. *Radiology* 1992;185:759–62

7. Monteagudo A, Timor-Tritsch I, Sharma S. Early and simple determination of chorionic and amniotic type in multifetal gestations in the first 14 weeks by high frequency transvaginal ultrasound. *Am J Obstet Gynecol* 1994;170:824–9

8. Hill LM, Chenevey P, Hecker J, Martin JG. Sonographic determination of first trimester twin chorionicity and amnionicity. *J Clin Ultrasound* 1996;24:305–8

9. Bessis R, Papiernik E. Echographic imagery of amniotic membranes in twin pregnancies. In Gedda L, Parisi P, eds. *Twin Research. 3. Twin biology and multiple pregnancy*. New York: Alan R Liss, 1981: 183–7

10. Finberg HJ. The 'twin peak' sign: reliable evidence of dichorionic twinning. *J Ultrasound Med* 1992;11:571–7

11. Sepulveda W, Sebire NJ, Hughes K, Odibo A, Nicolaides KH. The lambda sign at 10–14 weeks of gestation as a predictor of chorionicity in twin pregnancies. *Ultrasound Obstet Gynecol* 1996;7:421–3

12. Sepulveda W, Sebire NJ, Hughes K, Kalogeropoulos A, Nicolaides KH. Evolution of the lambda or twin/chorionic peak sign in dichorionic twin pregnancies. *Obstet Gynecol* 1997;89:439–41

13. Botting BJ, Macdonald Davies I, Macfarlane AJ. Recent trends in the incidence of multiple births and associated mortality. *Arch Dis Child* 1987;62:941–50

14. Doherty JDH. Perinatal mortality in twins, Australia, 1973–1980. *Acta Genet Med Gemellol* 1988;37:313–19

15. Chen CJ, Wang CJ, Yu MW, Lee TK. Perinatal mortality and prevalence of major congenital malformations of twins in Taipei city. *Acta Genet Med Gemellol* 1992;41:197–203

16. Pugliese A, Arsieri R, Patriarca V, Spagnolo A. Incidence and neonatal mortality of twins: Italy 1981–90. *Acta Genet Med Gemellol* 1994;43:139–44

17. Powers WF, Kiely JL. The risks confronting twins: a national perspective. *Am J Obstet Gynecol* 1994;170:456–61

18. Derom R, Vlietnick R, Derom C, Thiery M, Van Maele G, Van den Berghe H. Perinatal mortality in the East Flanders prospective twin survey. *Eur J Obstet Gynecol* 1991;41:25–6

19. Machin G, Bamforth F, Innes M, Minichul K. Some perinatal characteristics of monozygotic twins who are dichorionic. *Am J Med Genet* 1995;55:71–6

20. Sebire NJ, Snijders RJM, Hughes K, Sepulveda W, Nicolaides KH. The hidden mortality of monochorionic twin pregnancies. *Br J Obstet Gynaecol* 1997;104:1203–7

21. Luke B, Keith LG. The contribution of singletons, twins and triplets to low birth weight, infant mortality and handicap in the United States. *J Reprod Med* 1992;37:661–6

22. Dickey RP, Olar TT, Taylor SN, Curole DN, Rye PH, Matulich EM, Dickey MH. Incidence and significance of unequal gestational sac diameter or embryo crown–rump length in twin pregnancy. *Hum Reprod* 1992;7:1170–2

23. Achiron R, Blickstein I. Persistent discordant twin growth following IVF-ET. *Acta Genet Med Gemellol* 1993;42:41–4

24. Check JH, Chase JS, Nowrooki K, Goldsmith G, Dietterich C. Evidence that difference in size of fraternal twins may originate during early gestation: a case report. *Int J Fertil* 1992;37:165–6

25. Weissman A, Achiron R, Lipitz S, Blickstein I, Mashiach S. The first trimester discordant twin: an ominous prenatal finding. *Obstet Gynecol* 1994;84:110–14

26. Sebire NJ, Carvalho M, D'Ercole C, Souka A, Nicolaides KH. Intertwin disparity in fetal size in monochorionic and dichorionic twin pregnancies. *Obstet Gynecol* 1998;91:82–5

27. Benirschke K. Twin placenta in perinatal mortality. *N Y St J Med* 1961;61:1499–508

28. Schatz F. Eine besondere Art von einseitiger Polyhydramnie mit anderseitiger Oligohydramnie bei eineiigen Zwillingen. *Arch Gynakol* 1882;19:329

29. Benirschke K, Kim CK. Multiple pregnancy. *N Eng J Med* 1973;288:1276–84

30. Saunders NJ, Snijders RJM, Nicolaides KH. Twin–twin transfusion syndrome in the second trimester is associated with small inter-twin hemoglobin differences. *Fetal Diagn Ther* 1991;6:34–6

31. Saunders NJ, Snijders RJM, Nicolaides KH. Therapeutic amniocentesis in twin–twin transfusion syndrome appearing in the second trimester of pregnancy. *Am J Obstet Gynecol* 1992;166:820–4

32. Rosen D, Rabinowitz R, Beyth Y, Feijgin MD, Nicolaides KH. Fetal urine production in normal twins and in twins with acute polyhydramnios. *Fetal Diagn Ther* 1990;5:57–60

33. Rausen AR, Seki M, Strauss L. Twin transfusion syndrome. *J Pediatri* 1965;66:613–28

34. Abraham JM. Character of placentation in twins, as related to hemoglobin levels. *Clin Pediatr Phila* 1969;8,526–30

35. Tan KL, Tan R, Tan SH, Tan AM. The twin transfusion syndrome. Clinical observations on 35 affected pairs. *Clin Pediatr Phila* 1979;18:111–14

36. Danskin FH, Neilson JP. Twin-to-twin transfusion syndrome: what are appropriate diagnostic criteria? *Am J Obstet Gynecol* 1989;161:365–9

37. Hecher K, Ville Y, Snijders R, Nicolaides K. Doppler studies of the fetal circulation in twin–twin transfusion syndrome. *Ultrasound Obstet Gynecol* 1995 5:318–24

38. Sebire NJ, Hughes K, D'Ercole C, Souka A, Nicolaides KH. Increased fetal nuchal translucency at 10–14 weeks as a predictor of severe twin-to-twin transfusion syndrome. *Ultrasound Obstet Gynecol* 1997;10:86–9

39. Sebire NJ, Souka A, Carvalho M, Nicolaides KH. Inter-twin membrane folding as an early feature of developing twin-to-twin transfusion syndrome. *Ultrasound Obstet Gynecol* 1998;11:324–7

40. Elliott JP, Urig MA, Clewell WH. Aggressive therapeutic amniocentesis for treatment of twin–twin transfusion syndrome. *Obstet Gynecol* 1991;77:537–40

41. Reisner DP, Mahony BS, Petty CN, Nyberg DA, Porter TF, Zingheim RW, Williams MA, Luthy DA. Stuck twin syndrome: outcome in thirty-seven consecutive cases. *Am J Obstet Gynecol* 1993;169:991–5

42. Pinette MG, Pan Y, Pinette SG, Stubblefield PG. Treatment of twin–twin transfusion syndrome. *Obstet Gynecol* 1993;82:841–6

43. Peek MJ, McCarthy A, Kyle P, Sepulveda W, Fisk NM. Medical amnioreduction with sulindac to reduce cord complications in monoamniotic twins. *Am J Obstet Gynecol* 1997;176:334–6

44. Rodis JF, McIlveen PF, Egan JF, Borgida AF, Turner GW, Campbell WA. Monoamniotic twins: improved perinatal survival with accurate prenatal diagnosis and antenatal fetal surveillance. *Am J Obstet Gynecol* 1997;177:1046–9

45. Overton TG, Denbow ML, Duncan KR, Fisk NM. First-trimester cord entanglement in mono-amniotic twins. *Ultrasound Obstet Gynecol* 1999;13:140–2

46. Arabin B, Laurini RN, Van Eyck J. Early prenatal diagnosis of cord entanglement in monoamniotic multiple pregnancies. *Ultrasound Obstet Gynecol* 1999;13:181–6

47. Bajoria R. Abundant vascular anastamoses in monoamniotic versus diamniotic monochorionic placentas. *Am J Obstet Gynecol* 1998;179:788–93

48. Creinin M. Conjoined twins. In Keith LG, Papiernik E, Keith DM, Luke B. *Multiple Pregnancy.* Carnforth, UK: Parthenon Publishing, 1995;93–112

49. Spitz L. Conjoined twins. *Br J Surg* 1996;83:1028–30

50. Van Allen MI, Smith DW, Shepard TH. Twin reversed arterial perfusion (TRAP) sequence: study of 14 twin pregnancies with acardius. *Semin Perinatol* 1983;7:285–93

51. Moore TR, Galoe S, Bernischke K. Perinatal outcome of forty-nine pregnancies complicated by acardiac twinning. *Am J Obstet Gynecol* 1990;163:907–12

52. Quintero RA, Reich H, Puder KS, Bardicef M, Evans MI, Cotton DB, Romero R. Brief report: Umbilical cord ligation of an acardiac twin by fetoscopy at 19 weeks of gestation. *N Engl J Med* 1994;330:469–71

53. Ville Y, Hyett JA, Vandenbussche F, Nicolaides KH. Endoscopic laser coagulation of umbilical cord vessels in twin reversed arterial perfusion sequence. *Ultrasound Obstet Gynecol* 1994;4: 396–8

54. Pandya PP, Snijders RJ, Psara N, Hilbert L, Nicolaides KH. The prevalence of non-viable pregnancy at 10–13 weeks of gestation. *Ultrasound Obstet Gynecol* 1996;7:170–3

55. Sebire NJ, Thornton S, Hughes K, Snijders RJM, Nicolaides KH. The prevalence and consequence of missed abortion in twin pregnancies at 10–14 weeks of gestation. *Br J Obstet Gynaecol* 1997;104:847–9

56. Murphy KW. Intrauterine death in a twin: implications for the survivor. In Ward RH, Whittle M, eds. *Multiple Pregnancy*. London: RCOG Press, 1995: 218–30

57. Fusi L, MacParland P, Fisk N, Nicolini U, Wigglesworth J. Acute twin–twin transfusion: a possible mechanism for brain damaged survivors after intrauterine death of a monozygotic twin. *Obstet Gynecol* 1991;78:517–22

58. Jou HJ, Ng KY, Teng RJ, Hsieh FJ. Doppler sonographic detection of reverse twin–twin transfusion after intrauterine death of the donor. *J Ultrasound Med* 1993;12:307–9

59. MRC Working Party on children conceived by in vitro fertilisation. Births in Great Britain resulting from assisted conception, 1978–87. *Br Med J* 1990;300:1229–33

60. Burn J. Disturbance of morphological laterality in humans. *Ciba Found Symp* 1991;162:282–96

61. Baldwin VJ. Anomalous development of twins. In Baldwin VJ, ed. *Pathology of Multiple Pregnancy*. New York: Springer-Verlag, 1994:169–97

62. Sebire NJ, Sepulveda W, Hughes KS, Noble P, Nicolaides KH. Management of twin pregnancies discordant for anencephaly. *Br J Obstet Gynaecol* 1997;104:216–19

63. Ramos-Arroyo MA. Birth defects in twins: study in a Spanish population. *Acta Genet Med Gemellol* 1991;40:337–44

64. James WH. Concordance rates in twins for anencephaly. *J Med Genet* 1980;17:93–4

65. Guha-ray DK. Obstetric problems in association with anencephaly. A survey of 60 cases. *Obstet Gynecol* 1975;46:569–72

66. Evans MI, Goldberg JD, Dommergues M, Wapner RJ, Lynch L, Dock BS, Horenstein J, Golbus MS, Rodeck CH, Dumez Y, Holzgreve W, Timor Tritsch I, Johnson MP, Isada NB, Monteagudo A, Berkowitz RL. Efficacy of second-trimester selective termination for fetal abnormalities: international collaborative experience among the world's largest centers. *Am J Obstet Gynecol* 1994;171:90–4

67. Johnson SP, Sebire NJ, Snijders RJM, Tunkel S, Nicolaides KH. Ultrasound screening for anencephaly at 10–14 weeks of gestation. *Ultrasound Obstet Gynecol* 1997;9:14–16

68. Rogers JG, Voullaire L, Gold H. Monozygotic twins discordant for trisomy 21. *Am J Med Genet* 1982:11:143–6

69. Flannery DB, Brown JA, Redwine FO, Winter P, Nance WE. Antenatally detected Klinefelter's syndrome in twins. *Acta Genet Med Gemellol* 1984;29:529–31

70. Dallapiccola B, Stomeo C, Ferranti B, DiLecce A, Purpura M. Discordant sex in one of three monozygotic triplets. *J Med Genet* 1985;22:6–11

71. Perlman EJ, Stetten G, Tuck-Muller CM, Farber RA, Neuman WL, Blakemore KJ, Hutchins GM. Sexual discordance in monozygotic twins. *Am J Obstet Gynecol* 1990;37:551–7

72. Cuckle H. Down's syndrome screening in twins. *J Med Screen* 1998;5:3–4

73. Noble PL, Snijders RJM, Abraha HD, Sherwood RA, Nicolaides KH. Maternal serum free beta-hCG at 10 to 14 weeks in trisomic twin pregnancies. *Br J Obstet Gynaecol* 1997;104: 741–3

74. Sebire NJ, Snijders RJM, Hughes K, Sepulveda W, Nicolaides KH. Screening for trisomy 21 in twin pregnancies by maternal age and fetal nuchal translucency thickness at 10–14 weeks of gestation. *Br J Obstet Gynaecol* 1996;103:999–1003

75. Sebire NJ, Noble PL, Odibo A, Malligiannis P, Nicolaides KH. Single uterine entry for genetic amniocentesis in twin pregnancies. *Ultrasound Obstet Gynecol* 1996;7:26–31

76. Appelman Z, Caspi B. Chorionic villus sampling and selective termination of a chromosomally abnormal fetus in a triplet pregnancy. *Prenat Diagn* 1992;12:215–17

77. Christiaens GCML, Oosterwijk JC, Stigter RH, DeutzTerlouw PP, Kneppers ALJ, Bakker E. First-trimester prenatal diagnosis in twin pregnancies. *Prenat Diagn* 1994;14:51–5

78. Jorgensen FS, Bang J, Tranebjaerg L, Berge LN, Eik Nes SH, Schwartz M. Early prenatal direct gene diagnosis of cystic fibrosis in a twin pregnancy and subsequent selective termination. *Prenat Diagn* 1994;14:149–52

79. Brambati B, Tului L, Baldi M, Guercilena S. Genetic analysis prior to selective fetal reduction in multiple pregnancies: technical aspects and clinical outcome. *Hum Reprod* 1995;10:818–25

80. Sebire NJ, Noble PL, Psarra A, Papapanagiotou G, Nicolaides KH. Fetal karyotyping in twin pregnancies: selection of technique by measurement of fetal nuchal translucency. *Br J Obstet Gynaecol* 1996;103:887–90

81. Sebire NJ, Snijders RJM, Santiago C, Papapanagiotou G, Nicolaides KH. Management of twin pregnancies with fetal trisomies. *Br J Obstet Gynaecol* 1997;104:220–2

82. Abbas A, Johnson MR, Bersinger N, Nicolaides KH. Maternal serum alpha-fetoprotein in multifetal pregnancies before and after fetal reduction. *Br J Obstet Gynaecol* 1994;101:1561

83. Kiely J, Kleinman JC, Kiely M. Triplets and higher order multiple births. Time trends and infant mortality. *Am J Dis Child* 1992;146:862–8

84. Petterson B, Nelson KB, Watson L, Stanley F. Twins, triplets, and cerebral palsy in births in Western Australia in the 1980s. *Br Med J* 1993;307:1239–43

85. Yokoyama Y, Shimizu T, Hayakawa K. Prevalence of cerebral palsy in twins, triplets and quadruplets. *Int J Epidemiol* 1995;24:943–8

86. Evans MI, Dommergues M, Wapner RJ, Lynch L, Dumez Y, Goldberg JD, Zador IE, Nicolaides KH, Johnson MP, Golbus MS. Efficacy of transabdominal multifetal pregnancy reduction: collaborative experience among the world's largest centers. *Obstet Gynecol* 1993;82:61–6

87. Sebire NJ, Sherrod C, Abbas A, Snijders RJM, Nicolaides KH. Preterm delivery and growth restriction in multifetal pregnancies reduced to twins. *Hum Reprod* 1997;12:173–5

88. Nicolaides KH, Brizot M, Patel F, Snijders R. Comparison of chorionic villus sampling and amniocentesis for fetal karyotyping at 10–13 weeks' gestation. *Lancet* 1994;344:435–9

89. Bass HN, Oliver JB, Srinivasan M. Persistently elevated AFP and AChE in amniotic fluid from a normal fetus following the demise of its twin. *Prenat Diagn* 1986;6:33–5

90. Streit JA, Penick GD, Williamson RA, Weiner CP, Benda JA. Prolonged elevation of alphafetoprotein and detectable acetylcholinesterase after death of an anomalous twin fetus. *Prenat Diagn* 1989;9:1–6

91. Grau P, Robinson L, Tabsh K, Crandall BF. Elevated maternal serum alpha-fetoprotein and amniotic fluid alpha-fetoprotein after multifetal pregnancy reduction. *Obstet Gynecol* 1990;76:1042–5

92. Seppälä M, Ruoslahti E. Alpha fetoprotein: physiology and pathology during pregnancy and application to antenatal diagnosis. *J Perinat Med* 1973;1:104–13

93. Blakemore K, Baumgarten A, Schoenfeld-Dimaio M, Hobbins JC, Mason EA, Mahoney MJ. Rise in maternal serum α-fetoprotein concentration after chorionic villus sampling and the possibility of isoimmunization. *Am J Obstet Gynecol* 1986;155:988–93

94. Johnson MR, Abbas A, Nicolaides KH. Maternal plasma levels of human chorionic gonadotropin, oestradiol and progesterone before and after fetal reduction. *J Endocrinol* 1994;143:309–12

95. Abbas A, Johnson MR, Chard T, Nicolaides KH. Maternal plasma concentrations of insulin-like growth factor binding protein-1 and placental protein 14 in multifetal pregnancies before and after fetal reduction. *Hum Reprod* 1995;10:207–10

96. Lipitz S, Reichman B, Paret G, Modan M, Shalev J, Serr DM, Mashiach S, Frenkel Y. The improving outcome of triplet pregnancies. *Am J Obstet Gynecol* 1989;161:1279–84

97. Kingsland CR, Steer CV, Pampiglione JS. Outcome of triplet pregnancies resulting from IVF at Bourn Hallam 1984–1987. *Eur J Obstet Gynecol Reprod Biol* 1990;34:197–203

98. Seoud MAF, Kruithoff C, Muasher SJ. Outcome of triplet and quadruplet pregnancies resulting from in vitro fertilization. *Eur J Obstet Gynecol Reprod Biol* 1991;41:79–84

99. Melgar CA, Rosenfeld DL, Rawlinson K, Greenberg M. Perinatal outcome after multifetal reduction to twins compared with nonreduced multiple gestations. *Obstet Gynecol* 1991;78:763–6

100. Porreco RP, Burke S, Hendrix ML. Multifetal reduction of triplets and pregnancy outcome. *Obstet Gynecol* 1991;78:335–9

101. Bollen N, Camus M, Tournaye H, Vansteirteghem AC, Tournaye H, Devroey P. Embryo reduction in triplet pregnancies after assisted procreation: a comparative study. *Fertil Steril* 1993;60:504–8

102. Macones GA, Schemmer G, Pritts E, Weinblatt V, Wapner RJ. Multifetal reduction of triplets to twins improves perinatal outcome. *Am J Obstet Gynecol* 1993;169:982–6

103. Check JH, Nowroozi K, Vetter B, Vetter B, Rankin A, Dietterich C, Schubert B. The effects of multiple gestation and selective reduction on fetal outcome. *J Perinat Med* 1993;21:299–302

104. Boulot P, Hedon B, Pelliccia G, Peray P, Laffargue F, Viala JL. Effects of selective reduction in triplet gestation: a comparative study of 80 cases managed with or without this procedure. *Fertil Steril* 1993;60:497–503

105. Sebire NJ, D'Ercole C, Sepulveda W, Hughes K, Nicolaides KH. Effects of reduction from trichorionic triplets to twins. *Br J Obstet Gynaecol* 1997;104:1201–3

106. Vauthier-Brouzes D, Lefebvre G. Selective reduction in multifetal pregnancies: technical and psychological aspects. *Fertil Steril* 1992;57:1012–16

107. Timor-Tritsch IE, Peisner DB, Monteagudo A, Lerner JP, Sharma S. Multifetal pregnancy reduction by transvaginal puncture: evaluation of the technique used in 134 cases. *Am J Obstet Gynecol* 1993;168:799–804

108. Lynch L, Berkowitz RL, Chitkara U, Alvarez M. First-trimester transabdominal multifetal pregnancy reduction: a report of 85 cases. *Obstet Gynecol* 1990;75:735–8

109. Berkowitz RL, Lynch L, Lapinski R, Bergh P. First trimester transabdominal multifetal pregnancy reduction: a report of two hundred completed cases. *Am J Obstet Gynecol* 1993;169:17–21

110. Tabsh KMA. Transabdominal multifetal pregnancy reduction: report of 40 cases. *Obstet Gynecol* 1990;75:739–41

111. Tabsh KMA. A report of 131 cases of multifetal pregnancy reduction. *Obstet Gynecol* 1993;82:57–60

112. Shalev J, Frenkel Y, Goldenberg M, *et al.* Selective reduction in multiple gestations: pregnancy outcome after transvaginal and transabdominal needle-guided procedures. *Fertil Steril* 1989;52:416–21

113. Lipitz S, Reichman B, Uval J, Shalev J, Achiron R, Barkai G, Lusky A, Mashiach S. A prospective comparison of the outcome of triplet pregnancies managed expectantly or by multifetal reduction to twins. *Am J Obstet Gynecol* 1994;170:874–9

114. Rennie JM. Perinatal management at the lower margin of viability. *Arch Dis Child* 1996;74:F214–18

Index